MARCH OF DIMES NURSIN

Diabetes in Pregnancy

3rd Edition

Jo M. Kendrick, MSN, RNC, CDE

Editor
Rita Reis Wieczorek, EdD, RN, PNP, FAAN

Consulting Editor
Margaret Comerford Freda, EdD, RN, CHES, FAAN
Professor
Department of Obstetrics, Gynecology and Women's Health
Albert Einstein College of Medicine
Montefiore Medical Center
Bronx, New York

6.8 contact hours for RNs

.45 CEUs for CNMs
(CEUs expire 10/15/05)

33-1806-03 2/05
ISBN 0-86525-096-0

Library of Congress Cataloging-in-Publication Data

Kendrick, Jo. M.

Diabetes in pregnancy. – 3rd ed. / Jo M. Kendrick ; editor, Rita Reis Wieczorek ; consulting editor, Margaret Comerford Freda.

p. cm.

Includes bibliographical references.

ISBN 0-86525-096-0

1. Diabetes in pregnancy—Nursing. I. Wieczorek, Rita Reis. II. Freda, Margaret Comerford. III. Title.

[DNLM: 1. Pregnancy in Diabetes—nursing. 2. Obstetrical Nursing.]
RG580.D5P46 2004
618.3—dc21
2003046477

Published by:
March of Dimes
Education & Health Promotion

The mission of the March of Dimes Birth Defects Foundation is to improve the health of babies by preventing birth defects and infant mortality. To achieve this end, the Foundation funds programs of community service, advocacy, research and education. Part of our educational objective includes producing high-quality, low-cost education resources for health care providers, including March of Dimes nursing modules, assessment tools designed to enhance the skills of professionals who work with pregnant women and videos and brochures to help providers communicate key reproductive health messages to clients.

Some March of Dimes publications may, on occasion, contain controversial views. All such statements and opinions are the sole responsibility of the authors and do not reflect an endorsement by the March of Dimes or the editors unless expressly stated.

March of Dimes materials reflect current scientific recommendations at time of publication. These recommendations may change. Please check marchofdimes.com for updated information.

To order additional copies of this or any March of Dimes nursing module or to request a free March of Dimes continuing education catalog, call 800-367-6630.

For more information on March of Dimes nursing modules, contact:

March of Dimes
Education & Health Promotion
1275 Mamaroneck Avenue
White Plains, NY 10605
Phone: 914-997-4609
E-mail: profedu@marchofdimes.com
Web site: marchofdimes.com/nursing

TABLE OF CONTENTS

TABLE OF CONTENTS

TABLE OF CONTENTS

TABLE OF CONTENTS

Editor's Acknowledgements

Special thanks to author Jo M. Kendrick, MSN, RNC, CDE for making her knowledge available to nurses and health care providers through the publication of this module.

We also gratefully acknowledge the following reviewers who so generously shared their expertise:

Patricia Andronica, MS, RN, NPP, CDE
Diabetes Education Program Coordinator
Suffolk County Department of Health Services
Hauppauge, New York

Marie Luerssen RN, NP, CDE
Clinical Coordinator
Diabetes in Pregnancy Program
North Shore University
Manhasset, New York

Preface

March of Dimes nursing modules provide quality continuing education for nurses who deliver services to mothers and infants in a variety of health care settings. Recent years have seen dramatic changes in the world. All segments of society have been affected, altering our patterns of thinking, our actions and reactions. Technological advances have changed medical and nursing practice. Changing demographics have created new opportunities for providers to serve child-bearing families of diverse cultural back-grounds.

The March of Dimes recognizes the need to incorporate new, practical information and theoretical knowledge into nursing practice. To meet this challenge and promote excellent care for mothers and infants, the March of Dimes regularly convenes its Nurse Advisory Council to evaluate the nursing modules, to determine their direction and to recommend development of new titles addressing vital issues confronting nurses today.

General Information

Nursing modules are self-directed learning monographs written by expert nurses for nursing professionals who provide prenatal or perinatal care. Each module addresses a specific topic and provides practical clinical information. Topics range from preconception to the neonatal period and cover changes that occur during the transition from intrauterine to extrauterine life; care of the pregnant woman and her fetus; the labor and delivery period; care of the postpartum woman and her neonate; and current and future critical perinatal health problems. Each module provides background information and caregiving standards to meet these issues and addresses assessment of risk, stabilization of the client and emergency care.

Nursing modules do not supplant didactic educational and clinical experiences. Rather, they provide registered nurses with information to enhance their baseline skills. Differential experiences of the learner may require various levels of guidance to apply the materials to practice; for modules that deal with advanced practice topics, clinical application may initially require close supervision.

Module Format

Each nursing module includes several interrelated components and sections. *Cognitive Objectives* are rooted in the factual nature of each module. *Expected Practice Outcomes* stem from the clinical implications of these facts. *Key Concepts* facilitate identification of major points. The *Pre-/Postinstructional Measurement* assesses learner knowledge of the topic before and after module completion. *Clinical Application* emphasizes and provides reinforcement for clinical aspects of the material and allows transfer and implementation by the learner in a specific clinical setting. *Group Discussion Items* provide additional input from other learners and allow further exploration of cognitive and clinical objectives. *Supplementary Materials* provide annotated descriptions of multimedia resources to further enhance the module topic.

Getting the Most from the Module

To make the best use of a nursing module, first read the *Cognitive Objectives, Expected Practice Outcomes* and *Key Concepts* and answer and correct the *Pre-/Postinstructional Measurement.* Then read the module and complete the *Clinical Application.* If the module is being used in a group setting, the facilitator will arrange a meeting to discuss the *Clinical Application* and *Group Discussion Items.* As needed, review the *References* and *Supplementary Materials* to reinforce the module content and its utilization in clinical practice. Finally repeat the *Pre-/Postinstructional Measurement* to assess learning.

Evaluation

An evaluation is inserted in the module. Participants should remove and complete the evaluation, fold and staple it to reveal the postage-paid portion and post it in a U.S. mailbox. (Note: Group study participants may give the completed evaluation to their facilitator following the study session. Independent study takers may submit the completed evaluation directly to the March of Dimes; see the *Independent Study Application* for specific instructions.) Ongoing analysis of evaluations provides valuable data that enables the March of Dimes to offer the best possible continuing education for nurses.

Continuing Education Credit

This continuing education activity was approved by the New York State Nurses Association, an accredited approver by the American Nurses Credentialing Center's Commission on Accreditation. **It has been approved for 6.8 contact hours for registered nurses.**

American Nurses Credentialing Center/New York State Nurses Association approval applies only to the nursing education activity and does not indicate approval or endorsement of any commercial product used as part of the activity.

The March of Dimes is also approved as a continuing education provider by the State of California Board of Registered Nursing, Provider #CEP-11444.

This module is also approved for .45 continuing education units (CEUs) for certified nurse-midwives (CNMs) by the American College of Nurse-Midwives (ACNM) (program #2003/087). ACNM approval expires 10/15/05. CNMs should verify the module's approval status at marchofdimes.com/nursing if used after the expiration date.

To qualify for continuing education credit, participants must successfully complete the nursing module via **independent study** or **facilitated group study** as part of a hospital or other agency program, workshop, grand rounds or conference.

Independent Study

To receive continuing education credit for independent study, each participant must:

1. Be a registered nurse or certified nurse-midwife.
2. Complete the module, including the *Pre-/Postinstructional Measurement* and *Clinical Application.*
3. Take the *Independent Study Test* and complete the *Independent Study Application.*
4. Complete the module evaluation (self-mailer).
5. Submit the completed *Independent Study Application* and the module evaluation to: March of Dimes Nursing Modules, 1275 Mamaroneck Avenue, White Plains, NY 10605

The March of Dimes will notify participants of test results within 8 weeks of receiving the test. Participants with scores of 70 percent or higher will receive a certificate of completion; participants with scores less than 70 percent will be offered a second attempt to pass the test.

Independent study tests and applications are also available on the March of Dimes Web site at marchofdimes.com/nursing.

Facilitated Group Study

(Workshop/Grand ounds/Conference)

A facilitated group study requires facilitation by a qualified registered nurse. A facilitated group study may occur as an in-service education program, a workshop or nursing grand rounds, or may be a portion of a larger conference or educational meeting. To receive continuing education credit for facilitated group study, each participant must:

1. Be a registered nurse or certified nurse-midwife.
2. Complete the module before the facilitated group study, including the *Pre-/Post-instructional Measurement* and *Clinical Application.*
3. Participate in the facilitated group study.
4. Provide first and last name and mailing address to receive a certificate of completion.

The facilitator must:

1. Be a registered nurse or certified nurse-midwife.
2. Arrange time and location for the group study.
3. Facilitate discussion on the content of the module as well as the *Clinical Application* and *Group Discussion Items.*
4. Register as a group study facilitator by sending an e-mail to certificate@marchofdimes.com with facilitator name, organization name, mailing address and telephone number.
5. After receiving a confirmation e-mail reply, register the group study and participants and print certificates online at the Nursing Module Certificate Center. The e-mail confirmation will provide the Center's URL; required registration information includes module title; study date, location and facilitator; and participant names and addresses.
6. Distribute certificates of completion to participants.

Note: If a nursing module is used as part of a larger conference activity approved for continuing education credit, and continuing education credit is to be awarded for a facilitated group study on the nursing module, use the following formula to calculate the appropriate amount of credit: The number of contact hours/CEUs approved for the conference minus the number of contact hours/CEUs counted for the facilitated group study time plus the number of contact hours/CEUs approved for the module. See the following chart for an example:

Description	Credits
Full-day conference approved for 7 contact hours	7.0
Minus 1 hour for the facilitated group study using *Diabetes in Pregnancy,* 3rd Edition	-1.0
Plus 6.8 hours approved for the facilitated group study on *Diabetes in Pregnancy,* 3rd Edition	+ 6.8
Equals the total number of contact hours awarded for the conference plus the facilitated group study	**= 12.8**

For additional information, contact March of Dimes Education & Health Promotion:

Telephone	914-997-4609
Fax	914-997-4501
E-mail	profedu@marchofdimes.com
Web site	marchofdimes.com/nursing

About This Module

This module provides perinatal nurses with pertinent information to guide comprehensive nursing care and education of women with pregestational diabetes before conception and during the perinatal period. The module also presents education and intervention strategies for the care of women with gestational diabetes. The module addresses nursing management of complications of diabetes in pregnancy, as well as neonatal considerations.

March of Dimes
Saving babies, together®

Diabetes in Pregnancy, 3rd Edition
Facilitated Group Study Participant Roster

Facilitator______________________________ **Date**______________

Location____

Group study facilitators may use this sign-in sheet to record participant attendance.

	First Name	Last Name	Mailing Address	City	State	ZIP
1						
2						
3						
4						
5						
6						
7						
8						
9						
10						
11						
12						
13						
14						
15						
16						
17						
18						
19						
20						

AUTHOR

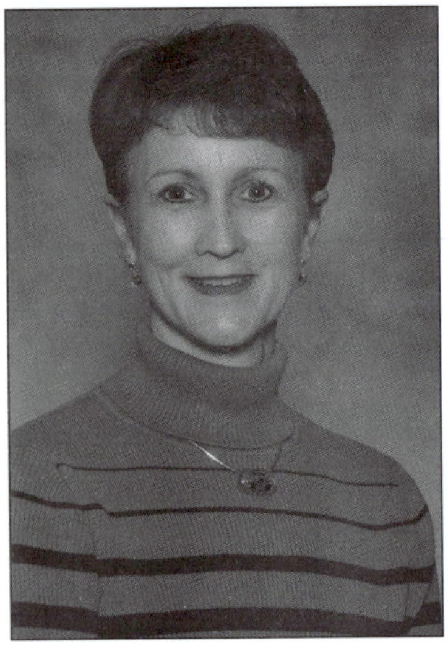

Jo M. Kendrick

BSN, University of Southern Mississippi, Hattiesburg, Mississippi

MSN, University of Tennessee College of Nursing, Knoxville, Tennessee

Jo M. Kendrick is Coordinator of the Perinatal Diabetes Program at the University of Tennessee Medical Center in Knoxville, Tennessee. She is also a women's health nurse practitioner in the Department of Obstetrics and Gynecology, Division of Maternal/Fetal Medicine at the University of Tennessee Medical Center. She serves as a Clinical Instructor in the Graduate School of Medicine for the University of Tennessee, Adjunct Clinical Instructor for the University of Tennessee College of Nursing and Clinical Assistant Professor for the Vanderbilt School of Nursing in Nashville, Tennessee. She is a member of the Association of Women's Health, Obstetric and Neonatal Nursing (AWHONN), the AWHONN Consulting Group, the American Diabetes Association (ADA) and Sigma Theta Tau. Ms. Kendrick is certified as a women's health nurse practitioner through the National Certification Corporation and as a certified diabetes educator from the National Certification Board for Diabetes Educators. She has served on the editorial board of the *Journal of Obstetric, Gynecologic and Neonatal Nursing*, serves on the board of the *Journal of Perinatal and Neonatal Nursing* and is a reviewer for *MCN, The American Journal of Maternal/Child Nursing.* Ms. Kendrick has published extensively in the area of women's health and diabetes and presents locally and nationally.

Ms. Kendrick has no real or perceived conflicts of interest related to this nursing module.

NURSING MODULE ORDER FORM

I ____

A ____

F ____

C ______________________________________ State ______ Zip ______________

F ______________________________ Fax (_____) ______________________________

E ____

(... ship to address)

Pl ____

wi ____

____

______________________________________ State ______ Zip ______________

______________________________ Fax (_____) ______________________________

____

ITE[M]		QUANTITY	PRICE EACH	TOTAL
33-[...]	[...]vention and Intervention, 2nd Edition		$20	
33-[...]	[...] Pregnancy, 2nd Edition		$20	
33-1610-01	The Art and Science of Labor Support		$20	
33-805-97	Assessment of Risk in the Term Newborn		$20	
33-720-00	Breastfeeding the Healthy Newborn: A Nursing Perspective		$20	
33-779-97	Breastfeeding the Infant with Special Needs		$20	
33-1905-04	Care of the Multiple-Birth Family: Postpartum Through Infancy		$20	
33-1904-04	Care of the Multiple-Birth Family: Preconception Through Postpartum		$20	
33-1656-02	Cultural Competence in the Care of Childbearing Families		$20	
33-1806-03	Diabetes in Pregnancy, 3rd Edition		$20	
33-1433-00	Discharge and Follow-Up of the High-Risk Preterm Infant		$20	
33-1520-01	Embryonic and Fetal Evaluation During Pregnancy		$20	
33-1751-02	Genetic Issues for Perinatal Nurses, 2nd Edition		$20	
33-676-00	Hemodynamic Monitoring of the Critically Ill Obstetric Patient		$20	
33-804-99	High-Risk Antepartal Home Care		$20	
33-900-98	High-Risk Pregnancy: Chronic Medical Conditions		$20	
33-891-97	Hypertensive Disorders of Pregnancy		$20	
33-1902-04	Interviewing by the Perinatal Nurse		$20	
33-1547-01	Loss and Grieving in Pregnancy and the First Year of Life: A Caring Resource for Nurses		$20	
33-675-00	The Mature Gravida: Pregnancy at Age 35 and Older		$20	
33-910-98	Nursing Assessment of the Pregnant Woman		$20	
33-1906-04	Obstetrical Emergencies for the Perinatal Nurse, 2nd Edition		$20	
33-1828-03	Perinatal and Neonatal Ethics: Facing Contemporary Challenges		$20	
33-1216-99	Perinatal Impact of Alcohol, Tobacco and Other Drugs		$20	
33-1859-04	Postpartum Care		$20	
33-1680-00	Preconception Health Promotion: A Focus on Women's Wellness		$20	
33-1451-00	Pregnancy: Psychosocial Perspectives, 3rd Edition		$20	
33-806-99	The Premature Infant: Nursing Assessment and Management		$20	
33-1805-03	Preterm Labor: Prevention and Nursing Management, 3rd Edition		$20	
33-1755-02	Package 1: Perinatal Care of the Low-Risk Woman		$85	
33-1922-04	Package 2: Neonatal Care		$102	
33-1756-02	Package 3: Perinatal Care of the High-Risk Woman		$187	
33-1757-02	Package 4: Psychosocial Issues		$119	

Method of Payment: *(Payment must accompany orders from individuals.)*

☐ Check – Payable to March of Dimes ☐ Visa ☐ American Express ☐ Master Card ☐ Discover

☐ Purchase Order #________________ Account Number ____________________ Exp. Date ____________

Marketing/Media Code ____________________ Signature ______________________________

SUBTOTAL	
SALES TAX* (CA only)	
SHIPPING (see back side of form)	
TOTAL	

All orders less than $50.00 must be prepaid. Prices are subject to change without notice.

**Sales/Use Tax: We are required by law to collect your state's sales/use tax on all orders. If claiming tax exemption, please attach a copy of your state sales tax exemption certificate. Currently applies to sales in CA only. States subject to change without notice.*

MARCH OF DIMES NURSING MODULE ORDER FORM

March of Dimes
Saving babies, together®

P.O. Box 932852
Atlanta, GA 31193-2852
Phone: 800-367-6630
Outside U.S.: 770-280-4115
Fax: 770-280-4116
Email: mod@pbd.com (for POs only)

Please use this form when submitting orders.

Standard Shipping & Handling Charges*

ORDER TOTAL	S&H CHARGE
$1 – $75	$5.95
$76 – $499	17%
$500 – $999	15%
Over $1,000	12%

Overnight, 2nd-day and same-day shipments: Call 1-800-367-6630 for rates.

Foreign shipments: Call 1-800-367-6630 for rates; must be prepaid in U.S. dollars.

All orders outside the U.S. must be prepaid.

*S&H charges subject to change without notice.

Please allow 2 weeks for delivery from the date we receive your order.

Fold Line

PLACE
POSTAGE
HERE

March of Dimes
Saving babies, together®

March of Dimes Fulfillment Center
P.O. Box 932852
Atlanta, GA 31193-2852

Fold Line

Pre-Packaged Nursing Modules

Designed to meet the ongoing educational needs of nurses working in maternal and infant health

15% savings over individual module purchase

Package 1: Perinatal Care of the Low-Risk Woman
Item # 33-1755-02 — $85

- The Art & Science of Labor Support
- Interviewing by the Perinatal Nurse
- Nursing Assessment of the Pregnant Woman
- Postpartum Care
- Preconception Health Promotion

Package 2: Neonatal Care
Item # 33-1922-04 — $102

- Assessment of Risk in the Term Newborn
- Breastfeeding the Healthy Newborn
- Breastfeeding the Infant with Special Needs
- Care of the Multiple-Birth Family: Postpartum Through Infancy
- Discharge and Follow-Up of the High-Risk Preterm Infant
- The Premature Infant: Nursing Assessment and Management

Package 3: Perinatal Care of the High-Risk Woman
Item # 33-1756-02 — $187

- Care of the Multiple-Birth Family: Pregnancy and Birth
- Diabetes in Pregnancy, 3rd Edition
- Embryonic & Fetal Evaluation During Pregnancy
- Genetic Issues for Perinatal Nurses, 2nd Edition
- Hemodynamic Monitoring of the Critically Ill Obstetric Patient
- High-Risk Antepartal Home Care
- High-Risk Pregnancy: Chronic Medical Conditions
- Hypertensive Disorders of Pregnancy
- The Mature Gravida: Pregnancy at Age 35 and Older
- Obstetrical Emergencies for the Perinatal Nurse, 2nd Edition
- Preterm Labor: Prevention and Nursing Management, 3rd Edition

Package 4: Psychosocial Issues
Item # 33-1757-02 — $119

- Abuse During Pregnancy, 2nd Edition
- Adolescent Pregnancy, 2nd Edition
- Cultural Competence in the Care of Childbearing Families
- Ethical Decision Making for Perinatal Nurses
- Loss & Grieving in Pregnancy and the First Year of Life
- Perinatal Impact of Alcohol, Tobacco and Other Drugs
- Pregnancy: Psychosocial Perspectives, 3rd Edition

COGNITIVE OBJECTIVES

Upon completion of this module, the learner will be able to:

1. Identify the significance of diabetes in pregnancy.
2. Determine insulin requirements in each trimester.
3. Discuss the impact of metabolic alterations on diabetes management in pregnancy.
4. Review appropriate methods for determining fetal well-being in pregnant women with pregestational and gestational diabetes.
5. Define education guidelines for pregnant women with pregestational and gestational diabetes.
6. Describe nursing management strategies for antepartum, intrapartum and postpartum care of women with diabetes.
7. Determine caloric requirements for metabolic management of pregnant women with diabetes.
8. List potential complications of maternal diabetes in the mother and infant.
9. Recognize signs and symptoms of diabetic ketoacidosis and appropriate nursing interventions for management.
10. Discuss psychosocial issues for pregnant women with diabetes.
11. Educate women with a history of gestational diabetes on appropriate follow-up testing criteria and diagnostic thresholds for type 2 diabetes mellitus and impaired fasting glucose or impaired glucose tolerance.
12. Identify risk factors for development of gestational diabetes and early testing.
13. List the screening and diagnostic thresholds for gestational diabetes.
14. Discuss nursing strategies for the care of pregnant women with vascular complications of diabetes during the antepartum and intrapartum periods.
15. Describe types of human insulin and their action appropriate for use during pregnancy.
16. Explain the role of self-monitoring of blood glucose in the care of pregnant women with diabetes.
17. Describe the glycemic thresholds for plasma and venous capillary blood.

EXPECTED PRACTICE OUTCOMES

The learner who meets the objectives and understands the key concepts of this module can be expected to:

1. Identify risk factors for the development of gestational diabetes and identify women who should be tested early in pregnancy.
2. Perform a systematic review of diabetes management in women with pregestational diabetes.
3. Provide education regarding all aspects of diabetes for women with pregestational and gestational diabetes.
4. Understand and treat hypoglycemia during the intrapartum period.
5. Identify risk factors for the development of diabetic ketoacidosis and recommend appropriate nursing interventions.
6. Outline appropriate fetal surveillance techniques for monitoring antenatal diabetes.
7. Identify women with gestational diabetes who require insulin initiation.
8. Provide counseling for follow-up of diabetes in the postpartum period.
9. Provide perinatal nursing care for women with vascular complications of diabetes.

KEY CONCEPTS

The material in this module will help the learner understand the following concepts:

1. Euglycemia during the preconception period reduces the risk that a woman with diabetes will spontaneously miscarry or deliver an infant with a congenital defect.

2. Pregnancy outcomes in women with diabetes are improved with strict metabolic control.

3. Fetal risk and infant morbidity are related to the level of maternal hyperglycemia.

4. Normal metabolic changes of pregnancy result in a diabetogenic state that significantly impacts diabetes management.

5. Risk status for gestational diabetes should be determined early in pregnancy and testing performed, if indicated.

6. Psychosocial issues affect self-care and adherence to management plans in women with pregestational and gestational diabetes.

7. Insulin sensitivity decreases with advancing gestation, requiring higher dosages of insulin to achieve euglycemia.

8. The presence of vascular disease in women during pregnancy increases the risk of higher perinatal morbidity and mortality.

9. A history of gestational diabetes mellitus increases the risk for development of overt type 2 diabetes in women.

PRE-/POSTINSTRUCTIONAL MEASUREMENT

Select the best response to each of the following questions. Check your answers with the key.

1. Type 2 diabetes mellitus is most often associated with:
   A. *An immune response that destroys the beta cells of the pancreas*
   B. *Auto-antibodies that develop in response to an environmental factor*
   C. *A genetic predisposition that produces symptoms before 20 years of age*
   D. *A pancreatic secretory defect that results in an inadequate supply of insulin*

2. Which metabolic adaptation to pregnancy increases during the later weeks of pregnancy?
   A. *Use of amino acids for hepatic gluconeogenesis*
   B. *Cellular sensitivity to glucose*
   C. *Breakdown of fatty tissue*
   D. *Anabolic activity*

3. When teaching a pregnant woman with diabetes mellitus about care during episodes of vomiting, the nurse should include instructions to:
   A. *Assess the urine for ketones twice a day*
   B. *Monitor blood glucose levels every 2 hours*
   C. *Discontinue insulin injections until vomiting subsides*
   D. *Drink sugar-free beverages regardless of blood glucose level*

4. When diabetic ketoacidosis is identified in a pregnant woman, the nurse should prepare to administer:
   A. *Fluids*
   B. *Electrolytes*
   C. *Oxygen therapy*
   D. *Subcutaneous insulin*

5. When teaching a woman to perform self blood glucose monitoring, it is most essential that the nurse:
   A. *Have the woman perform the procedure*
   B. *Demonstrate the procedure to a family member*
   C. *Give the woman written instructions about the procedure*
   D. *Discuss the relationship of diet and exercise to blood glucose*

6. To minimize the risk of hypoglycemia when breastfeeding, the nurse would teach a woman with diabetes mellitus taught to:
   A. *Exercise daily*
   B. *Eat a snack just before breastfeeding*
   C. *Decrease her daily calorie intake by 500 calories*
   D. *Use oral hypoglycemics, rather than insulin, while breastfeeding*

7. The nurse recognizes that a pregnant woman with diabetes is at risk for ketoacidosis when the woman:
   A. *Exercises excessively*
   B. *Takes too much insulin*
   C. *Experiences an infection*
   D. *Demonstrates a fluid volume excess*

8. When obtaining a patient history, which assessment is a risk factor related to gestational diabetes mellitus?
   A. *Caucasian race*
   B. *Age <25 years*
   C. *Family history of diabetes*
   D. *Weight <100 pounds*

9. For a woman with pregestational type 1 diabetes mellitus, insulin requirements will:
   A. *Decrease as the fetus produces insulin*
   B. *Increase sharply during organogenesis*
   C. *Double the prepregnancy dose by term*
   D. *Remain constant until the third trimester*

10. The significance of the increasing incidence of pregnant women with diabetes mellitus is that:
    A. *Diabetes precipitates the onset of obesity.*
    B. *Perinatal morbidity is higher in pregnancies complicated by diabetes.*
    C. *Most women with diabetes are diagnosed during the preconception period.*
    D. *Specific populations can account for the majority of the increase in diabetes.*

11. As part of antepartal care, which component is essential for all pregnant women with diabetes regardless of the type of diabetes or the presence of complications?
    A. *Insulin therapy*
    B. *Medical nutrition therapy*
    C. *Weight reduction program*
    D. *Strenuous physical exercise*

12. Before providing psychosocial support for a woman with diabetes, it is important for the nurse to understand that:
    A. *Empowerment of women with diabetes is the key to positive pregnancy outcomes.*
    B. *Women with gestational diabetes have greater anxiety levels than women who have pregestational diabetes.*
    C. *The level of glycemic control is directly related to the level of hostility in women with pregestational diabetes.*
    D. *Women with pregestational diabetes generally have acceptable glycemic control because of developed coping abilities.*

13. Infants born to mothers with diabetes often develop hypoglycemia after birth. To limit this complication, the nurse's initial action should be to:
    A. *Dry and warm the infant.*
    B. *Administer oxygen via a mask.*
    C. *Initiate an intravenous glucose infusion.*
    D. *Encourage breastfeeding or administer a glucose feeding.*

Answers to Pre-/Postinstructional Measurement

1.D 2.C 3.B 4.A 5.A 6.B 7.C 8.C 9.C 10.B 11.B 12.A 13.A

Diabetes in Pregnancy, 3rd Edition

Diabetes in pregnancy, whether pregestational or gestational, presents a challenge for the perinatal nurse.

Jo M. Kendrick

Introduction

Diabetes in pregnancy is a complex health care problem requiring a comprehensive, multidisciplinary approach to ensure a healthy outcome for both the woman and infant. Ideally, care for women with pre-existing diabetes should begin prior to conception to optimize perinatal outcome. Perinatal nurses caring for women with diabetes are challenged to provide care and education that incorporates diabetes management principles into obstetric care during all phases of childbearing, from preconception through the postpartum period. This care and education should be culturally sensitive and individualized to meet the physical and psychosocial needs of the childbearing woman.

The module addresses preconception nursing care and considerations of women with pre-existing diabetes, as well as nursing management strategies and care considerations for pregnant women with pregestational and gestational diabetes during the antepartum, intrapartum and postpartum periods.

Incidence and Significance

The prevalence of diabetes in the United States is increasing at an alarming rate and has already reached epidemic proportions. According to Centers for Disease Control and Prevention (CDC) data from the Behavioral Risk Factor Surveillance System (BRFSS), the incidence of diabetes (including gestational diabetes) increased from 4.9 percent in 1990 to 6.9 percent in 1999, representing an increase of 41 percent (Mokdad, Ford et al., 2001). Increases were noted in both males and females, all age groups, all ethnic groups, all educational levels and nearly all states. Prevalence varied by state, with Arizona reporting the lowest rate (2.9 percent) and Oklahoma reporting the highest (9.1 percent). Individuals aged 30 to 39 years had the highest increase (76 percent) in diabetes. These alarming statistics only reflect individuals with diagnosed diabetes and do not report on the prevalence of undiagnosed diabetes or people with impaired fasting glucose levels, which combined is estimated to account for another 18.8 million or 9.6 percent of the total U.S. population (Harris et al., 1998).

A contributing factor to increasing diabetes rates is the incidence of obesity. Obesity is defined as a body mass index (BMI) >30. Since 1991, obesity in the United States has risen by 57 percent, with approximately 17.9 percent of adults classified as obese (Mokdad et al., 2001b). Figures 1 and 2 depict diabetes and obesity trends among adults in the United States. The average weight of men in 1999 was 84.3 to 85.0 kg, and 68.5 to 68.7 kg for women, representing an increase in average weight from 76.2 kg in 1998 to 76.7 kg in 1999 (Mokdad, Ford et al., 2001). These trends have led to an increase in the incidence of diabetes in pregnancy in all ethnic and racial groups across the United States. Table 1 presents the diabetes rate in women by race/ethnicity per 1,000 births, both inside and outside the United States. Another contributing factor to the increasing rate of diabetes in the United States is immigration of women who have a higher rate of diabetes (Harris et al., 1998).

Perinatal morbidity and mortality are higher in pregnancies complicated by diabetes. Table 2 lists potential complications for the mother and infant. The risk of these outcomes may be reduced by intensive metabolic management and comprehensive obstetric care by health care providers.

Perinatal morbidity and mortality are higher in pregnancies complicated by diabetes.

Figure 1. Diabetes and Gestational Diabetes Trends Among Adults in the U.S., BRFSS 1990, 1995 and 2000

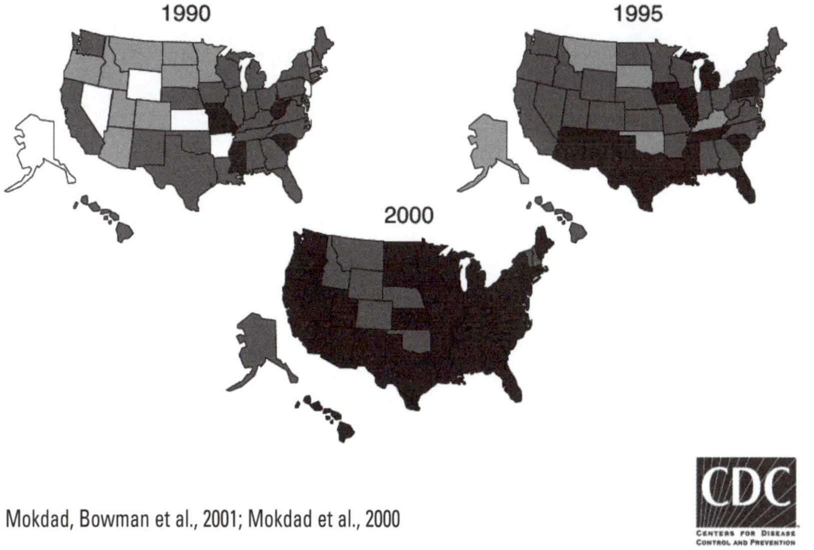

From Mokdad, Bowman et al., 2001; Mokdad et al., 2000

Figure 2. Obesity Trends Among U.S. Adults, BRFSS, 1991, 1995 and 2000

(*BMI ≥ 30, or ~ 30 lbs overweight for 5'4" woman)

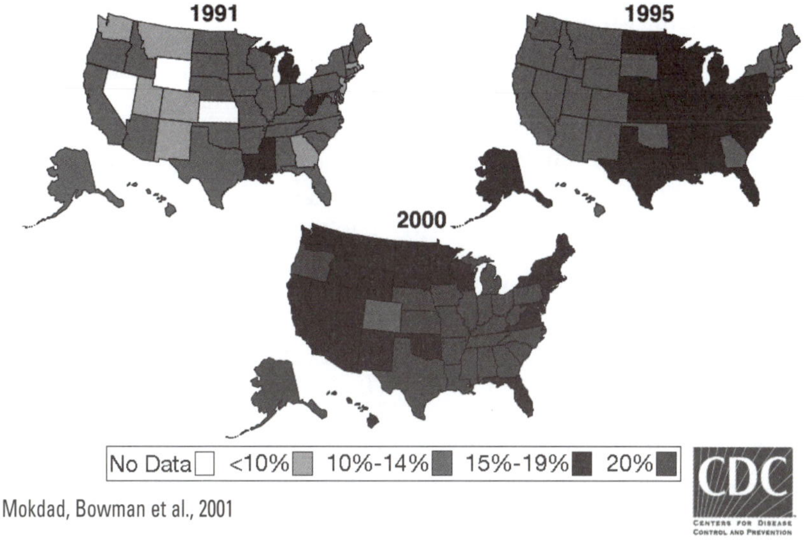

From Mokdad, Bowman et al., 2001

Table 1. Maternal Diabetes Rate per Race/Ethnicity

Race/Ethnicity	Adjusted Rate in the United States	Adjusted Rate outside the United States
Non-Hispanic		
White	24.3	23.0
Black	26.6	33.4
Hispanic		
Mexican	31.3	25.7
Puerto Rican	36.2	41.4
Cuban	24.3	21.4
Central or South America	21.3	24.3
American Indian/Alaskan Native	53.0	42.1
Asian/Pacific Islander		
Chinese	28.6	27.1
Japanese	27.7	15.6
Hawaiian	32.7	33.2
Filipino	29.9	32.0
Asian Indian	34.0	50.3
Korean	16.1	16.1
Samoan	17.7	31.0
Vietnamese	19.5	19.4
TOTAL ALL RACES/ ETHNICITIES	**25.0**	**26.4**

Adapted from CDC, 1998

Definition and Classification of Diabetes Mellitus

Diabetes mellitus is a chronic metabolic disease characterized by hyperglycemia as a result of limited or no insulin production, deficient insulin action or a combination of the two (Expert Committee on the Diagnosis and Classification of Diabetes Mellitus, 2003). Diabetes results in abnormalities in the metabolism of carbohydrates, proteins and fats, leading to the development of chronic hyperglycemia which, in turn, causes tissue damage. Diabetes is divided into two broad categories —type 1 and type 2—that are differentiated by their primary underlying etiology.

Type 1 diabetes is characterized by autoimmunity directed at the beta cells of the pancreas, resulting in absolute insulin deficiency (Ratner, 2001). This disorder is usually initially diagnosed in individuals <30 years of age, but it may develop at any age. Individuals with type 1 diabetes depend on exogenous insulin to sustain life and prevent the development of ketoacidosis (Ratner, 2001). Acute symptoms of hyperglycemia precede the diagnosis of type 1 disease and include polyuria, polydipsia and significant weight loss. If undetected and untreated, type 1

Table 2. Perinatal Morbidity and Mortality in Pregnancy Complicated by Diabetes

Maternal	Neonatal
Hypoglycemia	Macrosomia
Ketoacidosis	Stillbirth
Pyelonephritis	Intrauterine growth retardation
Pregnancy induced hypertension	Respiratory distress syndrome
Preterm labor	Asphyxia
Polyhydramnios	Hypoglycemia
Exacerbation of chronic complications	Polycythemia
Retinopathy	Hyperbilirubinemia
Nephropathy	Hypocalcemia
Gastroparesis	Hypomagnesemia
Neuropathy (autonomic)	Congenital defects
Cardiovascular disease	Birth injuries
Spontaneous abortion	Prematurity
Cesarean section	
Operative delivery	

diabetes can lead to coma and death (Ratner, 2001).

Type 2 diabetes, the most prevalent form, is characterized by a combination of insulin resistance and inadequate insulin production (Expert Committee on the Diagnosis and Classification of Diabetes Mellitus, 2003). Individuals with type 2 diabetes may be asymptomatic for a prolonged period of time because the degree of hyperglycemia is insufficient to result in clinical symptoms, but is sufficient enough to result in end organ damage. The average length of time from the development to the diagnosis of type 2 diabetes is 6.5 years (Matthews, 1999). Most cases of type 2 diabetes are diagnosed in individuals over the age of 30, but recent findings show that diabetes increased by 9.1 percent in 18- to 29-year-olds and 69.9 percent in 30- to 39-year-olds from 1990 to 1998 (Mokdad et al., 2001b). In contrast to type 1 diabetes, obesity predominates type 2 diabetes and contributes to its development. Individuals with type 2 diabetes are not ketosis prone. Type 2 diabetes may require exogenous insulin, but it often can be treated successfully with diet, exercise or oral hypoglycemic medications.

Diabetes in pregnancy is categorized into two groups: pre-existing diabetes, which includes women with type 1 or 2 disease, and women who develop diabetes during pregnancy, called gestational diabetes mellitus (GDM). GDM is defined as any degree of glucose intolerance with onset or first recognition during pregnancy (ADA, 2003d). Some women who are diagnosed with GDM early in pregnancy may have pre-existing diabetes; however, they are still classified as GDM until after pregnancy when diabetes diagnostic testing can be performed. Approximately 2 percent of women of childbearing age

The goal of preconception and early pregnancy nursing care is to obtain the lowest possible A1C without significant episodes of hypoglycemia.

have undiagnosed type 2 diabetes (Homko & Jornsay, 2001). The perinatal mortality rate in women with undiagnosed preexisting diabetes has been found to be six times higher than in women with GDM (Cundy et al., 2000).

Several classification systems have been designed as prognostic indicators for pregnancy outcome in women with pre-existing diabetes in pregnancy. The White classification system is the oldest and incorporates risk factors such as duration of diabetes, age at onset and presence of vascular complications to predict pregnancy outcome (White, 1949). However, this system does not consider the level of glycemia or include women with gestational diabetes, so it is used primarily for descriptive purposes. Pederson developed a classification system based on five signs—ketoacidosis, pyelonephritis, pregnancy-induced hypertension, self-neglect and limited prenatal care—which, if present, indicate a poorer prognosis (Pedersen & Anderson, 1974). A more recent classification system, introduced by Buchanan and Coustan (1995), includes diabetes type, glycemic control and presence of vascular complications. Gestational diabetes is also included for a subset of women with fasting normoglycemia (<105 mg/dL, diet controlled, $GDMA_1$) and fasting hyperglycemia (>105 mg./dL, insulin requiring, $GDMA_2$).

Preconception Care

Preconception Assessment and Management of Pregestational Diabetes

Women with diabetes should have prepregnancy counseling beginning at puberty and continuing throughout the reproductive life cycle (Jovanovic, 2000). This approach, combined with metabolic control, may minimize, if not eliminate, the risk of spontaneous abortion and delivering an infant with a congenital defect. Hemoglobin A1C (A1C), or glycosylated hemoglobin, is a laboratory determination that reflects the average blood glucose for the previous 4 to 6 weeks before the measurement. Women considering conception require intensive education and metabolic management by health care providers to maintain an A1C within 1 percent of normal (ADA, 2003g). Maintaining this level of glycemia before conception and during the period of organogenesis (6 to 8 weeks postconception) reduces the risk of congenital defects and spontaneous abortion to that of the non-diabetic population. Preconception nursing care should begin 3 to 6 months before the desired time of conception to allow for normalization of the A1C. In women who present in early pregnancy, the luxury of time is absent, and hospitalization is indicated to initiate strict metabolic control and intensive diabetes management to achieve euglycemia and reduce risk.

The preconception or pregnancy diabetes management team should be multidisciplinary to provide comprehensive care. Members should include the woman and her significant others, a perinatologist or obstetrician with high-risk experience, a diabetes specialist/endocrinologist, a nurse educator, subspecialists as indicated by chronic complications, a social worker or other psychosocial specialist with experience in dealing with individuals with diabetes, a dietician and others based on patient history. The March of Dimes nursing module *Preconception Health Promotion: A Focus for Women's Wellness* (Moos, 2003) discusses preconception care for women of childbearing age.

Holing and colleagues (1998) found that women with diabetes are aware that blood glucose levels should be optimized before conception; however, even with this knowledge, only 41 percent of pregnancies in women with diabetes are planned. Generally, women with diabetes who plan their pregnancies have higher incomes, more education and private health insurance, are happily married, are Caucasian, are less likely to use tobacco and receive care from an endocrinologist before conception (Holing, Beyer, Brown & Connell, 1998). Although pregnancy in women with diabetes is frequently not planned, women with diabetes are more likely than other women to seek prenatal care in the first trimester, regardless of race or ethnicity (CDC, 1998). The perinatal nurse must consider all of these factors when providing care for women preconceptionally.

Table 3. Elements of Effective Preconception Care

- Patient education regarding diabetes, pregnancy and family planning
- Assessment and education of diabetes self-management skills
- Obstetric and health care evaluation and laboratory testing
- Psychosocial assessment and interventions to reduce stress and improve adherence to the treatment regimen

From ADA, 2003g

The goal of preconception and early pregnancy nursing care is to obtain the lowest possible A1C without significant episodes of hypoglycemia (ADA, 2003g). Table 3 identifies elements of effective preconception care.

Preconception History

On the initial preconception visit, the nurse or physician should take a woman's complete health, obstetric and gynecologic history. Table 4 identifies information to be obtained in the history.

Table 4. Preconception History Information

- Diabetes type, age at onset, duration and disease course
- Acute complications, infection history, ketoacidosis and hypoglycemia, including the threshold for symptoms and hospitalization
- Chronic complications, including retinopathy with date of last dilated eye exam, nephropathy with date and results of previous 24-hour urine and metabolic profile, hypertension, cardiovascular disease with result of EKG or treadmill testing and autonomic or peripheral neuropathy
- History of other health care problems, including medications (over-the-counter and presciption) and treatment
- Current diabetic self-care practices, insulin dosage, oral antidiabetes medications, self-monitoring of blood glucose (SMBG), logging practices, medical nutrition therapy (MNT), use of alternative or complementary therapies and exercise
- Obstetric/Gynecologic history, including current and previous contraceptive use, menstrual history, history of infertility or polycystic ovarian syndrome and previous perinatal complications, including pregnancy-induced hypertension, polyhydramnios, macrosomia, intrauterine growth retardation, preterm birth, congenital defects, infections during pregnancy, route of delivery, labor complications, spontaneous abortions and neonatal complications
- Support systems, history of anxiety or depression and treatment, family relationships, financial support and work history
- Risk behaviors, including alcohol, tobacco and drug use

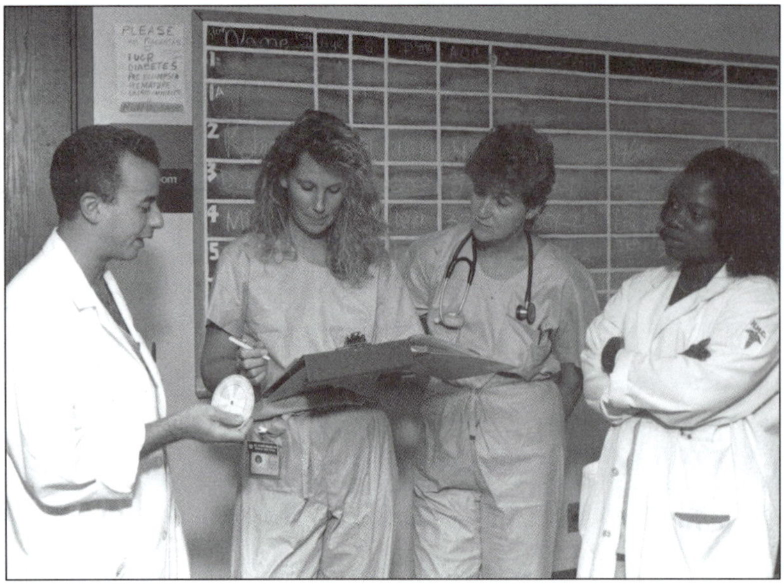

Acute Complication Assessment

Hypoglycemia
A fine balance of food intake, physical activity, insulin therapy and metabolic needs interplay to achieve normoglycemia in individuals with diabetes. Maintenance of euglycemia is the ultimate goal of diabetes management, but it is difficult to achieve and maintain. Most individuals have fluctuations in blood glucose, from low or hypoglycemic levels to high or hyperglycemic levels (Gonder-Frederick, 2001). However, frequent episodes of severe hypoglycemia may indicate poorly managed diabetes, lack of adherence to or understanding of the diabetes management plan, psychosocial dysfunction or hypoglycemia unawareness. The nurse should explore all of these areas to determine underlying etiology and the most appropriate treatment plan. The multidisciplinary health care team should determine the blood glucose level at which the symptoms of hypoglycemia occur, the symptoms usually exhibited and the mode of treatment. The team should also ensure that the woman has access to emergency carbohydrate or glucose tablets, an emergency hypoglycemia treatment kit and a person trained in its administration.

Hypoglycemia is defined as a blood glucose level of 70 mg/dL (3.9 mmol/L) or lower (Gonder-Frederick, 2001). The severity of hypoglycemia, however, is based on symptomatology ranging from mild symptoms, including lightheadedness, sweating, trembling, hunger, parasthesia, tachycardia, difficulty concentrating or pallor, to more severe symptoms, including confusion, lethargy or unconsciousness, rendering self-treatment difficult or impossible. Symptoms of hypoglycemia are individualized and can change over time as counterregulatory function becomes impaired. The autonomic nervous system provides the early warning signs of hypoglycemia as a result of hormonal counterregulation. Hormonal counterregulation causes the liver to release stored glucose and epinephrine, decreasing utilization of glucose and contributing to hepatic production of glucose.

Counterregulatory hormone production by the alpha cells of the pancreas diminishes after the first few years of diabetes in individuals with type 1 disease (Gonder-Frederick, 2001). At this point, epinephrine becomes the primary protection against hypoglycemia. This protective mechanism diminishes over time, leaving the woman with diabetes with few warning signs of hypoglycemia, a condition called hypoglycemia unawareness. Significant neuroglycopenia may result, in which the individual cannot initiate treatment due to impaired cognition. Neuroglycopenia may also result in emotional and behavioral changes, including anxiety, tension, irritation, anger, frustration, sadness, giddiness, euphoria, disinhibition, arguing, crying, resistance to treatment, aggression and inappropriate social/sexual behaviors (Gonder-Frederick, 2001). These behaviors may cause family members and loved ones significant distress, particularly when they are trying to treat the hypoglycemia in the face of aggression. Nurses play a significant role in supporting and educating the family on recognition and appropriate treatment of hypoglycemia.

Women with hypoglycemia unawareness should check their blood glucose levels frequently. Ongoing exploration and adjustment of the treatment plan minimizes episodes of hypoglycemia and may involve manipulating the diet, altering the amount or timing of the insulin dosage and altering activity. Nocturnal hypoglycemia should be avoided because the woman may not awaken with early symptoms. Checking a blood glucose level at bedtime and at 2:00 a.m. or 3:00 a.m. will assist in adjustment of insulin to prevent hypoglycemia and determine bedtime snacking requirements. Education should also include a warning that a second episode of hypoglycemia within 24 hours may be more dramatic due to a temporary deficit in epinephrine response (Heller & Cryer, 1991). Nurses should encourage all women with diabetes who take insulin, especially those with hypoglycemia unawareness, to wear identification jewelry.

Diabetic Ketoacidosis

Diabetic ketoacidosis (DKA) is a serious, acute complication. DKA results from insulin deficiency, increasing gluconeogenesis, decreased glucose utilization, increased lipolysis and increased ketogenesis, which causes hyperglycemia and ketoacidosis. Precipitating factors may include insufficient insulin, infection, severe stress, dehydration, nausea and vomiting, insulin pump failure, steroid administration and noncompliance. A history of several episodes of DKA warrants further nursing investigation to determine the underlying cause or multiple contributing factors. The nurse should educate the woman and her significant others about specific, preventive strategies and early recognition of signs and symptoms that warrant contacting a health care provider. Because the key to DKA management is prevention, early detection and aggressive treatment are critical. The woman should receive a psychosocial evaluation to identify stressors and coping mecha-

Table 5. Elements of Sick Day Management

- The woman should continue taking insulin. Dosage may need to be increased, even if she cannot tolerate the prescribed diet.
- The woman should check urine ketones every 4 to 6 hours during episodes of vomiting or fever. She should contact her health care provider when the results are moderate.
- The woman should check blood glucose levels every 2 to 3 hours during periods of excessive vomiting. She should notify her health care provider about levels >200 mg/dL.
- The woman should take antinausea medication as prescribed.
- To avoid dehydration, the woman should consume liquids equal to the carbohydrate content of the prescribed diet if solid foods are not tolerated. She should consume sweet beverages slowly. She should consume sugar-free beverages if blood glucose levels are >120 mg/dL.
- The woman should promptly report signs and symptoms of infection to her health care provider.

Retinopathy is the most frequently encountered diabetes-related chronic complication present during pregnancy.

nisms, and she should thoroughly understand how to manage diabetes during illness. Table 5 identifies elements of this "sick day management."

Chronic Complication Assessment

Retinopathy

A history of microvascular, macrovascular and neuropathic complications of diabetes increases perinatal morbidity and mortality. During the preconception period, the nurse should educate the woman and her family about the potential effects of pregnancy. Retinopathy is the most frequently encountered diabetes-related chronic complication present during pregnancy. Retinopathy usually progresses in an orderly fashion from mild nonproliferative, characterized by increased vascular permeability, to moderate and severe nonproliferative diabetic retinopathy (NPDR), characterized by vascular closure leading to proliferative diabetic retinopathy (PDR) (ADA, 2003c). PDR is characterized by neovascularization denoting new growth of blood vessels in the retina and posterior surface of the vitrous (ADA, 2003c). Vision is impaired due to edema and nonperfusion of the new capillaries. Retinal detachment can occur with contraction of the scarred tissue, producing severe and irreversible vision loss. Evidence of PDR requires laser photocoagulation before conception and continued surveillance during pregnancy.

Retinopathy prevalence is strongly related to duration of diabetes. Individuals with type 1 diabetes should have a dilated eye exam by an opthamologist 5 years after diagnosis, and then annually. Individuals with type 2 diabetes should have an eye exam on diagnosis of diabetes (because their diabetes may have been present several years before diagnosis), and then annually (ADA, 2003c). Nearly all individuals with type 1 diabetes and more than 60 percent of individuals with type 2 diabetes will have retinopathy after 20 years of diabetes (ADA, 2003c).

For unknown reasons, pregnancy accelerates the progression of retinopathy. A marked elevation in placental lactogen and other placental angiogenic factors that result in vessel proliferation in vivo may induce vascular changes in the retina and contribute to the progression of retinopathy in pregnancy (Rosenn & Miodovnik, 2000). Rapid normalization of blood glucose has been linked to retinopathy progression (Diabetes Control and Complications Trial [DCCT] Research Group, 1993; Rosenn & Miodovnik, 2000). Maternal hypertension has also been associated with retinopathy. Laser photocoagulation of PDR after conception is controversial; however, women with significant neovascularization are at great risk of retinal hemorrhage, and the benefit is greater than the risk in these women (Homko & Jornsay, 2001). Women who have untreated PDR may require a cesarean birth or laboring down (spontaneous pushing only) to avoid the Valsalva maneuver during second stage pushing. Background retinopathy can be managed by continued surveillance, because regression usually occurs after delivery.

Nephropathy

Women with type 1 diabetes of 20 years duration have a 40 percent to 50 percent chance of developing diabetic nephropathy, a 24-hour urinary protein excretion >300 mg/dL (Coonrod & Ernst, 2001). Occurrence in type 2 diabetes is much less common, reported at 5 percent to 10 percent, but nephropathy may be present at diagnosis, reflecting prolonged, undetected hyperglycemia (Coonrod & Ernst, 2001). Women with type 1 diabetes should be screened for albuminuria annually after 5 years of their disease, and women with type 2 diabetes should be tested annually after diagnosis because their disease may not have been precisely dated (ADA, 2003b). Microalbuminuria is defined as proteinuria between 30 mg/day and 300 mg/day from a 24-hour collection. Three methods are available for detecting microalbuminuria: a 24-hour urine collection with protein and creatinine clearance, an albumin-to-creatinine ratio in a random spot collection and a timed collection (ADA, 2003b). Transient elevations of albuminuria may occur secondary to illness, exercise or hyperglycemia, requiring repeat testing to confirm the diagnosis.

Nephropathy greatly affects perinatal mortality and morbidity in pregnancy, resulting in a higher incidence of preterm birth, cesarean birth, pregnancy-induced hypertension, worsened existing hypertension, edema, maternal anemia, intrauterine growth retardation and stillbirth (Rosenn & Miodovnik, 2000; Reece, Leguizamon & Homko, 1998; Star & Carpenter, 1998). The incidence of perinatal complications increases with the amount of proteinuria. Women who have microalbuminuria deliver prematurely 62 percent of the time, while those with overt nephropathy deliver premature infants 91 percent of the time (Ekbom et al., 2001). Women with microalbuminuria give birth to small-for-gestational-age infants at a rate of 4 percent, increasing to 45 percent in overt nephropathy (Ekbom et al., 2001). In addition, offspring of women with diabetes complicated by nephropathy have developmental delays and lower body weights than children born to women with diabetes without nephropathy (Biesenbach, Grafinger, Zazgornik & Helmut, 2000; Kimmerle et al., 1995). Women with proteinuria of <190 mg/day have a 7 percent chance of developing pregnancy-induced hypertension, increasing to 31 percent with proteinuria of 190 mg/day to 499 mg/day, and 38 percent with proteinuria of >500 mg/day (Combs et al., 1993). Pregnancy outcome can be improved with aggressive control of hypertension.

Angiotensin converting enzyme (ACE) inhibitors are the drugs of choice for delaying the progression of diabetic nephropathy but are contraindicated in pregnancy due to adverse fetal effects. However, their use in the preconception period (with contraception) may improve pregnancy outcome (Bar et al., 1999). Antihypertensive agents that may be used in pregnancy are methyldopa, calcium channel blockers and alpha adrenergic blockers to maintain a blood pressure of 130/80 (Rosenn & Miodovnik, 2000).

Most studies show that pregnancy does not alter the rate of decline in renal function, nor does pregnancy increase the risk for subsequent development of nephropathy. However, women with serum creatinine of >3 mg/dL and a creatinine clearance of <50 ml/min should be counseled to avoid pregnancy until after renal transplantation (ADA, 2003b).

Neuropathy

Diabetic neuropathy is a peripheral nerve dysfunction that encompasses a group of clinical and subclinical syndromes affecting sensory and autonomic pathways (Funnell & Feldman, 2001). An association between pregnancy and an increase in the prevalence of neuropathy has not been found (Rosenn & Miodovnik, 2000). The prevalence of neuropathy increases with the duration of diabetes and lack of glycemic control in individuals with type 1 and 2 disease. Hyperglycemia results in nerve glycosylation, hypoxia and accumulation of polyols in the nerve cells, leading to cofactor depletion with resulting nerve damage (DCCT, 1993). Individuals with peripheral neuropathy may also have diabetic autonomic neuropathy (DAN). While any body system may manifest DAN, pregnancy is negatively affected when the gastrointestinal or cardiovascular systems are involved.

Gastroparesis, or gastropathy, involves autonomic neuropathy of the viscera, resulting in decreased innervation of the stomach or intestines, which causes delayed gastric emptying and limited nutrient absorption. Delayed absorption of carbohydrates makes insulin adjustments of rapid acting insulin difficult, if not impossible. Symptoms described by patients with gastroparesis may result in malnourishment and include early satiety, weight loss, bloating, epigastric pain, nausea, vomiting and diarrhea. Maternal and fetal morbidity is high with this disorder due to the difficulty in maintaining adequate nutrition, which very often requires hospitalization and hyperalimentation. Diagnosing gastroparesis requires tests that evaluate and measure the neuromuscular activity of the stomach. Pharmacologic interventions include the use of metoclopramide before each meal and at bedtime, erthromycin to improve gastric emptying and domperidone, a promotility agent under review by the Food and Drug Administration (FDA). Anti-emetic administration may also help with control of nausea and vomiting, and loperamide may be given for diarrhea. Non-pharmacologic methods include smaller, more frequent meals, liquid nutrition and avoidance of high fiber and fatty foods (National Institute of Diabetes and Digestive and Kidney Diseases [NIDDK], 1999). A jejunostomy or parenteral nutrition are reserved for severe gastroparesis when all other methods fail.

Autonomic neuropathy directed at the cardiovascular system may result in orthostatic hypotension, cardiac denervation with a fixed heart rate and a risk for sudden painless myocardial infarction or an abnormal cardiovascular response to exercise (Funnell & Feldman, 2001). Orthostatic hypotension is a decrease in systolic blood pressure of more than 30 mm Hg, or a diastolic drop of more than 10 mm Hg within 2 minutes of standing from a supine position (Funnell & Feldman, 2001). Presyncopal episodes occur with patients describing symptoms of dizziness, tunnel vision, light-headedness, weakness and, eventually, syncope. Postural hypotension may be minimized by educating the patient to change positions slowly, to wear pressure stockings to decrease venous pooling and to sleep with the head of the bed elevated by 30 degrees (Funnel & Feldman, 2001). Hypovolemia can be avoided by increasing dietary sodium intake, achieving glycemic control and, in severe cases, administering mineralcorticoids such as fludrocortisone (Windebank & Feldman, 2001). Pregnancy already carries some risk of postural hypotension; additional safety precautions for the pregnant woman include having someone nearby during showering or bathing, avoiding extreme heat and maintaining adequate hydration.

Cardiac denervation is a fixed heart rate that does not increase in response to exercise, stress, breathing patterns or sleep (Funnell & Feldman, 2001). Diagnosis is made by testing for autonomic neuropathy or by obtaining an EKG during deep breathing, exercise or Valsalva (Funnell & Feldman, 2001). Lack of variation in the heart rate indicates nerve damage. This poses a threat to pregnancy, which requires an increase in plasma volume and cardiac output. Lack of heart rate variation is a contraindication to pregnancy.

Hypoglycemia unawareness may indicate autonomic neuropathy with ineffective production of epinephrine and glucagon in response to hypoglycemia. Use of long or intermediate acting insulin, with small doses of rapid acting insulin with meals, may control blood glucose levels more consistently and prevent hypoglycemic episodes. Continuous subcutaneous insulin infusion (CSII) therapy should also be considered in women with hypogloycemia unawareness.

Coronary Artery Disease

Coronary artery disease (CAD) is a macrovascular disease involving ateriosclerotic and atherosclerotic changes in moderate- to large-sized arteries and veins (Vinicor, 2001). The three major types of macrovascular disease in diabetes are coronary artery disease, cerebral vascular disease and peripheral vascular disease. The incidence of CAD is two to four times higher in patients with nephropathy than in those without (Homko & Jornsay, 2001). CAD carries significant risk of maternal mortality due to the impact of hemodynamic and cardiovascular changes associated with pregnancy (Rosenn & Miodovnik, 2000). Survival rates have improved in the last decade, but estimates are based on a small number of women. These rates may reflect improved obstetric and cardiovascular care or a decrease in conception in women who are advised against conception. Regardless, women with diabetic coronary artery disease are at great risk of an ischemic cardiac event or myocardial infarction during pregnancy and in the early postpartum period when cardiac output significantly rises. In addition, strict glycemic control in women with heart disease carries a risk of hypoglycemia with release of catecholamines that cause tachycardia and possible arrythmias, possibly leading to cardiac ischemia (Rosenn & Miodovnik, 2000).

Preconception care in women with diabetes of 10 years duration or in those with symptoms (angina or dyspnea) of cardiac disease should include an EKG, a stress test, a lipid profile and testing for microalbuminuria or albuminuria (ADA, 2003h). The preconception nursing history should include risk for cardiac disease (hyperlipidemia, smoking, family history and obesity). Women who have revascularized with normal exercise tolerance after coronary bypass grafting may proceed with pregnancy, but they must be aware that the hemodynamic tolerance of their cardiovascular system cannot be predicted (ADA, 2003g). All pregnant women with diabetes and coronary heart disease require intense surveillance by an endocrinologist, cardiologist and high-risk obstetrician or perinatologist.

Preconception Physical Examination

A careful physical examination during the preconception period should focus on the detection of vascular complications and other diabetes-related abnormalities. Blood pressure assessment should include evaluation for orthostatic changes that might indicate autonomic neuropathy. The nurse should take the blood pressure with the woman sitting, supine and immediately on standing, repeating at 1, 3 and 5 minutes. Symptoms of dizziness, tunnel vision, light-headedness or weakness with standing, and a documented decrease in the diastolic blood pressure of 10 mm Hg, or a 30 mm Hg decrease in the systolic pressure, indicate the need for autonomic function testing. The nurse should also assess the woman's pulse rate during position

No contraceptive options are specifically contraindicated for women with diabetes.

change. A fixed rate or minimal change with position change warrants further diagnostic testing. Systems are available to evaluate autonomic function. If these are not available, referral to a neurologist is warranted. Women with diabetes of 10 years duration or with symptoms of heart disease should also have an EKG and a stress test.

The nurse's skin assessment should include observation of injection sites for signs of lipohypertrophy, lipoatrophy, bruising, inflammation, erythema and correct rotation of injection sites. Evidence of lipohypertrophy indicates the need for selection of another body region for injections for at least 6 to 12 months to allow healing of the hypertrophic areas. Insulin absorption is diminished when injected into a hypertrophic area. Utilizing a new site may improve absorption, and the insulin dose may be reduced. The nurse should educate the woman about possible hypoglycemia. The nurse should also assess the skin of the extremities for corns, callus formation, nail fungus, thickened nails, dry skin, edema, poorly healing wounds and ulcers.

Deep tendon reflexes, muscle strength, position sense and temperature are also necessary components of the complete physical examination of women with diabetes (Feldman et al., 1994). Application of a tuning fork to the distal first metatarsal head assesses vibratory sensation. The nurse can also use a tuning fork to test for temperature sensation by placing the fork on the skin and asking the woman to describe the temperature (Funnell & Feldman, 2001). Vibration and monofilament testing assess pain and light touch sensation. Figure 3 shows the suggested sites for monofilament testing of the feet. The nurse can assess the woman's position sense by having her flex and extend her big toes and asking her to describe the position.

Loss of ankle reflexes, decreased tactile perception, loss of position sense and decreased vibration sensation indicate sensory neuropathy of small and large fibers (Funnell & Feldman, 2001). Absence of the dorsalis pedis and posterior tibialis pulses indicates the presence of peripheral vascular disease (Ahroni, 2001).

Filling time is measured by elevating the legs by 45 degrees for 1 minute and then dangling the legs over the side of the examining table and noting the time in seconds when the veins bulge

Figure 3. Sites for Monofilament Testing of the Feet (5.07 monofilament)

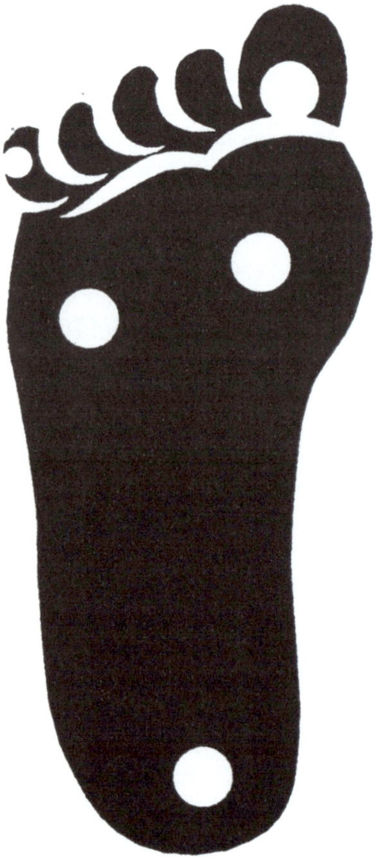

From Ahroni, 2001
Reprinted with permission

above the skin (Ahroni, 2001). Normal venous filling time in the feet is <20 seconds; >20 seconds is abnormal (Ahroni, 2001). Other signs of vascular insufficiency include hairless toes, shiny skin, atrophy of subcutaneous fat and thickened nails (Logan, 1993). The nurse should educate the woman about self-assessment and care of the feet. Table 6 identifies topics to be included in footcare education.

A nurse practitioner or physician should perform a complete gynecologic history and examination and obtain a pap smear and other cultures as indicated by history. Infertility is not more prevalent in women with diabetes, but the provider should identify and treat any abnormality that might inhibit fertility to enhance conception once preconception glycemic control is achieved. If conception is to be delayed, the provider and woman should explore contraceptive options. No contraceptive options are specifically contraindicated for women with diabetes (ADA, 2003g). Contraception with a low failure rate is essential for women whose diabetes is in poor control to prevent a pregnancy at great risk for spontaneous abortion or having an infant with a birth defect. The provider should obtain the woman's weight, blood pressure, glycemic control and fasting serum lipid levels for comparison before initiation of hormonal contraception (Kjos, 2000). For hormonal contraceptives, the nurse should recommend follow-up visits after the first cycle, and then every 3 to 4 months to assess the effect on blood pressure and metabolic parameters (Kjos, 2000). Lipids should be assessed annually in women with diabetes. Table 7 provides contraceptive options for women with diabetes.

Preconception Laboratory Assessment Table 8 identifies tests to be included in the preconception laboratory assessment. Other tests may be added based on the preconception history and physical examination.

Table 6. Foot Care Education

For proper foot care, the woman should:

- Inspect the tops, bottoms and sides of the feet and interdigital areas daily. Use a magnifying mirror, if necessary.
- Shake out shoes before putting them on and feel inside for irregularities or loose objects.
- Avoid going barefoot or wearing only socks. Use sunscreen on feet and wear footwear at the pool and beach.
- Wash and dry feet completely, especially between the toes.
- Avoid applying heat to the feet—from bathing or soaking or from any other heated application.
- Apply moisturizer that does not contain alcohol (alcohol can cause drying). Avoid application between the toes.
- Cut toenails straight across and file the edges smooth. Ask a family member, podiatrist or nurse to help if you have visual difficulties or cannot reach your feet.
- Do not self-treat corns, calluses or ingrown toenails.
- Wear well-fitted socks made of soft cotton, synthetic blend or wool.
- Seek care from a health care provider for any problems, such as fungal infections, poorly healing wounds, calluses, blisters cuts, or signs of infection.

From Ahroni, 2001

Table 7. Contraceptive Options for Women with Diabetes

Method	Failure Rate (Accidental Pregnancy Rate with Typical Use During the First Year)	Effect on Lipids and Carbohydrate Metabolism	Considerations and Risks
Barrier methods			
Condoms with foam (male)	14 percent	None	Less effective than other methods
Female condom	21 percent	None	May increase risk for urinary tract infections (UTIs) for women prone to UTIs
Diaphragm with spermicide	20 percent	None	May increast risk of UTIs
Cervical cap with spermidice	40 percent parous 20 percent nulliparous	None	May increase risk of UTIs
Oral contraceptives			
Combined estrogen/ progestin; low-dose monophasic or triphasic	5 percent	Minimal	May increase insulin requirement; should be closely monitored
Progestin only	5 percent	Minimal; avoid in breastfeeding or lactating women with GDM history (Kjos, 2000)	May increase insulin requirement; should be closely monitored
Combined estrogen/ progestin; high dose	5 percent	Moderate	Increased risk for thrombophlebitis, pulmonary embolism and cardiovascular disease
Intrauterine device	0.8 percent	None	Increased risk for pelvic infection
Injectable progestin	0.3 percent	Minimal in general population; unstudied in diabetes	Requires closer monitoring of blood glucose (BG) and metabolic profile
Combined injectable	0.1 percent to 0.4 percent	Minimal in general population; unstudied in diabetes	Requires closer monitoring of BG and metabolic profile
Norplant	.05 percent	Minimal in general population; unstudied in diabetes	Requires closer monitoring of BG and metabolic profile
Male sterilization or vasectomy	0.1 percent	None	Safest for women with vascular disease
Female sterilization or bilateral tubal	0.8 percent to 3.7 percent, depending on type	None	Surgical and anesthetic risk; may pose less risk than pregnancy

Adapted from Nelson et al., 2000

Table 8. Preconception Laboratory Assessment

- Complete blood count (CBC), electrolytes
- Glycosylated hemoglobin or hemoglobin A1C
- Urinalysis
- 24-hour urine for protein and creatinine clearance
- Thyroid profile, including antithyroid antibodies for women with type 1 diabetes, thyroid stimulating hormone and free thyroxine levels
- Fasting lipid profile (total cholesterol, high density lipoprotein [HDL], triglycerides and low density lipoproteins [LDL])
- Rubella immunity
- Blood type and Rh

Medical Nutrition Therapy Assessment

A medical nutrition therapy (MNT) assessment is another vital component of the preconception evaluation. It should be obtained after the history and physical examination to incorporate findings into the nutrition plan. Figures 4 and 5 provide examples of a nutrition history form and diet record that the woman may complete before the appointment or by the dietician or nurse during the appointment. MNT includes the use of individualized nutrition services to treat an illness or condition, incorporating personal preferences, culture, financial implications and the desire to change lifestyle habits to achieve nutritional goals (Franz, 2001). MNT provides the cornerstone of diabetes management for all diabetes types and replaces previously used terms such as diet, diet therapy or management. A registered dietician should explore the nutritional knowledge, cultural/ethnic preferences and overall lifestyle of the woman. Factors that affect nutrition therapy include the overall diabetes treatment program; laboratory data such as the A1C, blood glucose levels, metabolic panel and result of urinary albumin assessment; presence of vascular disease or other medical illness; medications; physical activity limitations; and use of complementary therapies.

Folate supplementation is recommended for the preconception period to decrease the risk of neural tube defects and can be accomplished by administration of a vitamin with 400 mcg of folate (Moos, 2003). Women who have preconception anemia should take iron supplements. If the woman's diet is calcium deficient, she should take additional calcium with vitamin D.

The nurse can evaluate eating patterns by obtaining a dietary recall or by having the woman complete a food record, including activity level and insulin regimen. Individualized MNT includes food/meal planning appropriate for the woman's lifestyle and diabetes management goals; education concerning diabetes and nutrition therapy and diabetes management; and nutrition goals (Franz, 2001). Caloric requirements are based on the woman's weight and activity level, with obese, sedentary women requiring approximately 20 kcal/kg; active women requiring 25 kcal/kg; and very active women requiring 30 kcal/kg (Franz, 2001). The meal plan should be integrated into the insulin regimen and daily activity to optimize metabolic control without excessive weight gain, which may occur in women with type 2 diabetes taking insulin for the first time. MNT for obese women with diabetes may include modest weight reduction strategies. Insulin sensitivity improves with weight loss and may reduce insulin requirements. Calories should be reduced by 500 kcal/day to allow for a 1-pound weight loss per week.

Folate supplementation is recommended for the preconception period to decrease the risk of neural tube defects and can be accomplished by administration of a vitamin with 400 mcg of folate.

Figure 4. Nutrition History

Name______________________ Date of birth__________ MD__________ Date__________

Diabetes type__________ Age @ diagnosis______________

Age______ Sex M F Height______ Weight______ Desired weight______

Highest weight__________ When?________ Lowest weight__________ When?__________

Weight loss/gain in past year________Why?________________________

Medication/Vitamin supplements	Dose

With whom do you live?______________________ Who shops for groceries?__________

Who cooks?______________ Occupation______________ Work hours__________

Describe any physical activity or exercise you do and how often you do it. ______________________

____

Meals eaten away from home	How often?	Where?
Breakfast		
Lunch		
Dinner		

Do you add salt to your food after cooking?______________ While cooking?______________

What beverages do you drink?______________________________

Do you drink alcohol?__________ What, how much and how often?______________________

____

Figure 5. Food Intake History

Breakfast

I don't eat breakfast. Yes No

I usually eat breakfast between ______________(earliest) and ______________(latest).

One breakfast I often eat is (food/portion): ______________________________

Another breakfast I sometimes eat is (food/portion): ______________________________

I eat breakfast ___________ days per week.

Mid-Morning Snack

I don't eat a mid-morning snack. Yes No

I usually eat a mid-morning snack between _______________(earliest) and_______________(latest).

One snack I often eat is (food/portion): ______________________________

Another snack I sometimes eat is (food/portion): ______________________________

I eat a mid-morning snack ____________days per week.

Lunch

I don't eat lunch. Yes No

I usually eat lunch between ____________ (earliest) and _______________(latest).

One lunch I often eat is (food/portion): ______________________________

Another lunch I sometimes eat is (food/portion):______________________________

I eat lunch _____________ days per week.

Afternoon Snack

I don't eat an afternoon snack. Yes No

I usually eat an afternoon snack between _______________(earliest) and ________________(latest).

One afternoon snack I often eat is (food/portion): ______________________________

Another afternoon snack I sometimes eat is (food/portion): ______________________________

I eat an afternoon snack ______days per week.

Evening Meal

I don't eat an evening meal. Yes No

I usually eat an evening meal between _______________(earliest) and ________________(latest).

One evening meal I often eat is (food/portion): ______________________________

Another evening meal I sometimes eat is (food/portion): ______________________________

I eat an evening meal ____________days per week.

Evening Snack

I don't eat an evening snack. Yes No

I usually eat an evening snack between _______________(earliest) and ________________(latest).

One evening snack I often eat is (food/portion): ______________________________

Another evening snack I sometimes eat is (food/portion): ______________________________

I eat an evening snack ____________days per week.

Psychosocial factors play an integral role in diabetes management due to the psychological and behavioral demands of the disease.

Amount and type of exercise should be evaluated and incorporated into the insulin regimen and eating pattern to avoid hypoglycemia. Exercise is an essential component of management of type 2 diabetes and has beneficial effects for individuals with type 1 diabetes, although an improvement in glycosylated hemoglobin has not been shown (ADA, 2003f). Exercise in individuals with micro- and macrovascular disease is contraindicated, due to risks outweighing benefits. Follow-up should occur periodically during the preconception period to re-evaluate and modify medical nutrition therapy and exercise goals, as indicated.

Psychosocial Assessment

Psychosocial factors play an integral role in diabetes management due to the psychological and behavioral demands of the disease (Delamater et al., 2001). Fifteen percent of individuals with diabetes have clinical depression and poorer glycemic control as a result of depression (Peyrot & Rubin, 1997; Lustman et al., 2000). Social support, particularly spousal, positively influences diabetes regimen adherence (Trief, Himes, Orendorff & Weinstock, 2001). Pouwer and colleagues (2001) found that evaluation of psychological well-being at outpatient visits had a positive impact on mood profile, although glycemic control was not influenced.

Identification and clarification of issues that may affect the woman's ability to manage her diabetes should be explored during the preconception period. A comprehensive psychosocial assessment may not be feasible due to time constraints; however, an initial, brief assessment (Table 9) may identify variables that warrant further exploration and possible referral to a mental health specialist. Psychosocial issues that warrant exploration include attitudes, beliefs and intentions; physical and emotional health status; skills; and family and community factors (Rubin & Napora, 2001).

Women with type 2 diabetes self-administering insulin for the first time may be apprehensive and may need family support, as well as support from the diabetes management team. Education that is sensitive to the woman's needs and concerns provides the foundation for her accepting injections.

Financial status and the possible burden of pregnancy and childcare should also be evaluated. A pregnant woman with pre-existing diabetes and vascular disease may require prolonged bedrest or hospitalization that prevents her from working, which may cause additional stress. The nurse should discuss with the woman the possibility and financial impact of neonatal intensive care for the infant due to prematurity, congenital defects or other electrolyte abnormalities. Consultation with a social worker may be indicated to evaluate possible resources for the family.

Self-Management Assessment

Self-monitoring of blood glucose is an important aspect of diabetes management. Individuals with diabetes who self-monitor daily, even though not frequently, have lower A1C levels than those who do not (Karter et al., 2001). The nurse should thoroughly review self-care practices to determine the woman's education needs and to help her attain preconception glycemic goals. The frequency of blood glucose testing and logging practices should be determined. Quality controls on the reflectance meter should be obtained, and the meter should be replaced if its performance is not optimal. A simultaneous blood draw for a laboratory determination of plasma glucose should be obtained and compared to

Table 9. Brief Psychosocial Assessment

Health Beliefs
On a scale of 1 (strongly disagree) to 10 (strongly agree), how much do you agree that:
1. You'll be healthier later in life if you control your diabetes now.
2. Changing your eating habits will help you control your diabetes.

Self-Efficacy
On a scale of 1 (confidence very low) to 10 (confidence very high), how confident do you feel about your ability to:
1. Manage your diabetes on a daily basis
2. Use a blood glucose meter to test your blood glucose level

Behavior Intentions
How often do you plan to:
1. Monitor blood glucose levels
2. Walk or do other exercise

Stress
1. Is having diabetes stressful for you?
2. What is most stressful about dealing with your diabetes?

Quality of Life
1. How is diabetes affecting the quality of your life?
2. On a scale of 1 (very unsatisfied) to 10 (very satisfied), are you satisfied with your quality of life?

Emotional Well-Being
1. Self esteem: How do you feel about yourself?
2. Depression: How often do you feel sad or tired or have low interest in life and things you used to enjoy?
3. Anxiety: Do you often feel nervous or on edge about your diabetes?
4. Eating disorder: How often do you eat too much or too little?

Family/ Social Support
How much do your family and friends help you care for your diabetes?

From Rubin & Napora, 2001
Reprinted with permission

the meter value to determine correlation. Meters that report plasma values from whole blood should be within 10 percent at glucose concetrations ranging from 30 mg/dL to 400 mg/dL (ADA, 1994). After teaching and demonstration, the nurse should observe the woman's technique for obtaining a blood glucose to determine deficits in performance. The nurse should review all aspects of insulin administration, including drawing up mixed-dose insulins, injection technique, site rotation, insulin storage and disposal of biohazardous waste. For women using a subcutaneous insulin pump, the nurse should review their equipment, determine the frequency of site change and rotation and observe their catheter placement technique. The nurse should assess the need for medical alert jewelry and encourage its use, if appropriate.

Women with type 2 diabetes previously controlled by oral antidiabetes agents must discontinue these medications during the preconception period and require comprehensive education regarding all aspects of insulin administration. The use of oral antidiabetes medications during pregnancy cannot be recommended due to limited study; however, one study of the use of glyburide in the second and third trimester of women with GDM showed some promise (Langer, Conway, Berkus, Xenaki & Gonzales, 2000).

Continuous glucose monitoring may help the woman and her provider make decisions regarding insulin, dietary intake, activity and exercise in the preconception period. The system provides multiple blood glucose readings via a subcutaneous port usually worn on the abdomen for 72 hours. The woman records insulin, food intake and activity. After 72 hours, the health care provider downloads and evaluates the information and adjusts the diabetes regimen, considering diurnal variations in blood glucose levels.

Preconception Education, Counseling and Follow-Up

The woman and her health care team should formulate a comprehensive, individualized and mutually agreed-upon plan for diabetes management during the preconception period. The team should educate and counsel the woman and her significant others based on their learning needs. Several sessions may be required using written materials, videos, practice sessions with return demonstrations and discussion. Group or individual sessions may enhance the learning process. Table 10 lists glycemic goals for therapy; Figure 6 provides a sample preconception education checklist.

Follow-up visits to assess attainment of metabolic control occur monthly, or more frequently if additional evaluation is needed, such as blood pressure assessment for women with vascular disease who require blood pressure monitoring, hypoglycemic unawareness or other health care problems. Frequent telephone contact may be necessary to evaluate blood glucose levels and to adjust insulin. Table 11 identifies elements of a follow-up visit.

Antepartum Care

Diabetes Management in Pregnancy: Pregestational and Gestational

Women with pre-existing diabetes ideally should have planned pregnancies when their metabolic control is optimal, but this is not usually observed. Women who have diabetes predating pregnancy require immediate attention to their disease and obstetric condition, particularly if they are in or near the period of organogenesis. Strict

Table 10. Preconception Glycemic Goals

Timing	Whole Blood	Plasma
Fasting	70 mg/dL to 100 mg/dL	80 mg/dL to 110 mg/dL
Pre-meal	70 mg/dL to 100 mg/dL	80 mg/dL to 110 mg/dL
1 hour post-meal	<140 mg/dL	<155 mg/dL
2 hours post-meal	<120 mg/dL	<135 mg/dL
Bedtime <120 mg/dL	<135 mg/dL	

From Jovanovic, 2000

Figure 6. Preconception Education Checklist

Name________________________ Date of birth______________ Age__________

Diabetes type__________________ Age @ diagnosis__________ Insulin dose______________

Blood pressure________ Height________ Weight __________

Urine: Protein____ Glucose_____ Ketones____ Educator______________________

The woman with diabetes desiring preconception control will demonstrate the following:

Expected Outcomes	Date
Understands diabetes, role of glucose and insulin transport	
Understands significance of hemoglobin A1C for spontaneous abortion and congenital defect. Hemoglobin A1C result Date	
Understands the effect pregnancy has on diabetes control, including the role of placental hormones	
Understands 24-hour urine and chemistry results, including potential complications of nephropathy/microalbuminuria during pregnancy, hypertension, pregnancy-induced hypertension, severe edema, bedrest, hospitalization, intrauterine growth restriction, preterm delivery and intrauterine fetal death.	
Understands the importance of eye examination before conception, with treatment and monitoring of retinopathy	
Uses a glucose meter, including quality controls	
Uses an autolancet to obtain a blood sample with appropriate disposal	
Understands the diabetes diet/diary and the role of exercise with safety guidelines	
Uses appropriate recording technique for blood glucose values and abnormal reactions	
Understands glycemic goals for treatment	
Knows onset and peak times of prescribed insulin	
Appropriately inspects and stores insulin	
Correctly draws up insulin (single and mixed)	
Identifies injection timing, injection sites, rotation and technique and appropriate syringe disposal	
Identifies signs and symptoms of hypoglycemia	
Knows about hypoglycemia unawareness and its potential risks	
Understands appropriate treatment of hypoglycemia with documented low (written guidelines)	
Has a support person who demonstrates knowledge of glucagon use and appropriate administration—provided Rx with two refills	
Identifies signs and symptoms of ketoacidosis and the importance of reporting persistent nausea/vomiting, illness, infection, persistent hyperglycemia or recurrent insulin reactions	
Understands the importance of checking ketones with blood glucose values >250 mg/dL	
Understands appropriate sick day management (written guidelines)	
Understands plan of care, visit schedule and follow-up lab testing	
Understands the significance of diabetes and development of long-term complications related to poor control	

Level of comprehension______________________ Learning impediments__________________

Family support______________ Previous education______________ Meter______________

Nurses play an integral role in caring for women with pregestational and gestational diabetes.

Table 11. Elements of a Follow-Up Visit

- Download meters and determine correlation to logged values to identify falsification, over-reporting or under-reporting.
- Address with the woman the underlying causes of low correlations, including depression, anxiety or the woman feeling she cannot achieve the standards for glycemia.
- Obtain glycosylated hemoglobin measurement at 6- to 8-week intervals until the desired goal is reached.
- Evaluate appropriate use of contraception at each visit to prevent conception before attainment of optimal glycemic control. Discontinue contraception when glycemic goals are reached; however, continue follow-up to ascertain maintenance of metabolic control.
- Continue nutritional and psychosocial assessments; refer to appropriate health care professionals, as indicated.

metabolic control is indicated to decrease the risk of spontaneous abortion or congenital defects. A comprehensive diabetes assessment and physical examination should be performed to determine if hospitalization is required or if the woman can be safely managed in an ambulatory setting, and to diagnose micro- or macrovascular abnormalities that affect pregnancy management.

Women with newly diagnosed gestational diabetes mellitus also require a thorough assessment and an individualized diabetes management plan. Comprehensive education is required to empower the woman and her family to understand, accept and incorporate the diabetes regimen into her daily life. Nurses play an integral role in caring for women with pregestational and gestational diabetes.

Metabolic Alterations of Pregnancy

Profound metabolic adaptations occur during pregnancy to meet maternal and fetal requirements. These changes allow continuous nutrient flow to the growing fetus, even though the mother intermittently feeds. Early pregnancy is characterized as an anabolic phase in which insulin production and sensitivity improve due to the hormonal influences of progesterone and estrogen. The hyperinsulinemic state in the first and early second trimester results in increased fat production and storage in preparation for the increased energy demands of later pregnancy. Exogenous insulin requirements may be reduced by 10 percent to 20 percent in women with type 1 diabetes by the end of the first trimester (Jovanovic, 2000). Episodes of hypoglycemia are more frequent in early pregnancy as a result of less predictable insulin requirements, nausea and vomiting.

The second half of pregnancy has been characterized as diabetogenic because of hyperglycemia in the face of hyperinsulinemia, the metabolic change that allows continuous flow of nutrients and glucose to the fetus. Insulin production increases dramatically in the latter half of pregnancy because of decreased insulin sensitivity resulting from the influence of pregnancy hormones that are insulin antagonistic—estrogen, progesterone, human placental lactogen (HPL), human chorionic somatomammotropin (HCS), cortisol and prolactin. Insulin requirements in pregnant women with type 1 and 2 diabetes increase by 50 percent to 60 percent, compared to their pre-pregnancy needs (Jovanovic, 2000).

Another metabolic alteration that affects the latter half of pregnancy is the rapid switch from carbohydrate to fat metabolism during periods of maternal fasting. Glucose and amino acids are reserved for the fetus during fasting while the pregnant woman utilizes lipids for energy. This lipolysis results in increased ketone production, which the mother does not buffer as well, increasing the risk of diabetic ketoacidosis in women with type 1 diabetes. Hepatic glucose production increases by 16 percent to 30 percent as a result of lipolysis, which generates production of glycerol, fatty acids and ketones. Glycerol drives gluconeogenesis (glucose production by the liver from precursors such as lactate and amino acids), while oxidation of fatty acids produces the fuel to support gluconeogenesis (Butte, 2000).

Screening and Diagnosis of Gestational Diabetes

Metabolic changes associated with pregnancy may result in glucose intolerance in women who are at risk. For high-risk women, screening is recommended between 24 and 28 weeks gestation. Table 12 identifies testing criteria for women at risk for developing GDM.

Table 12. Testing Criteria for Women at Risk for Developing GDM

- Age >25 years
- Family history of diabetes
- History of poor obstetric outcome
- History of abnormal glucose metabolism
- Obesity
- Member of high-risk racial/ethnic group
  - Hispanic
  - Native American
  - South or East Asian
  - African American
  - Pacific Islander

From ADA, 2003d

Only one criterion must be met to indicate the need for testing. Many physicians screen all women for GDM because most women exhibit at least one risk factor (American College of Obstetricians and Gynecologists [ACOG], 2001). Providers should screen women at higher risk for GDM development in the first trimester or at the first prenatal visit. Screening prior to the 24th week gestation should be considered for women with marked obesity, a history of GDM, glycosuria or a family history of diabetes (ADA, 2003d). If testing results are negative before 24 weeks gestation, screening should be repeated between 24 and 28 weeks gestation.

Testing for GDM occurs as a one- or two-step approach based on level of risk and economic factors. In the one-step approach, the diagnostic 3-hour oral glucose tolerance test (OGTT) is performed. The two-step approach, the preferred method in the United States, involves first performing the 1-hour glucose challenge test (GCT), followed by the diagnostic 3-hour OGTT in women who exceed the threshold for the GCT (ADA, 2003d). The GCT

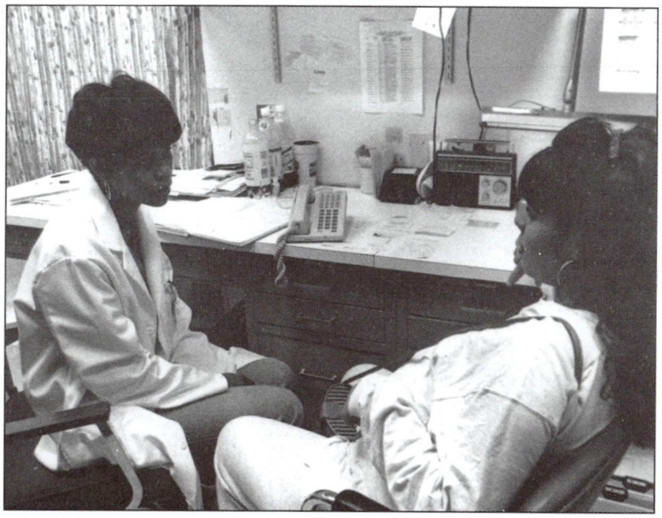

Insulin requirements in pregnant women with type 1 and 2 diabetes increase by 50 percent to 60 percent, compared to their pre-pregnancy needs.

Table 13. OGTT Diagnostic Thresholds

OGTT (100 g)	Plasma Value
Fasting blood sugar	95 mg/dL
1 hour	180 mg/dL
2 hours	155 mg/dL
3 hours	140 mg/dL

Two values above the plasma value threshold are diagnostic for GDM.

From ADA, 2003d

threshold plasma value of 140 mg/dL identifies approximately 80 percent of women with GDM, whereas a threshold of 130 mg/dL increases detection to 90 percent (ADA, 2003d). However, using the 130 mg/dL cutoff requires approximately 25 percent of women to have the OGTT, with only 15 percent requiring the OGTT if the 140 mg/dL is used. ACOG (2001) supports the use of either cutoff. A fasting plasma glucose level of >126 mg/dL is considered diagnostic for GDM and does not require oral glucose testing. A random plasma glucose of >200 mg/dL, when confirmed on another day, is also diagnostic for GDM. Women who exhibit these levels of hyperglycemia should have an A1C to estimate the length of time that hyperglycemia has existed. If the level is elevated, closer maternal and fetal surveillance should be instituted, by following guidelines for monitoring women with type 2 disease. Table 13 lists the diagnostic thresholds for the OGTT. The 75-g, 2-hour oral glucose tolerance test also is used for GDM diagnosis, using the same thresholds as the 100-g test and omitting the 3-hour blood draw value. The 100-g test has been well-validated for detection of maternal and infant risk, whereas the 75-g test has had minimal testing (ADA, 2003d).

Diagnosis of GDM requires meeting or exceeding two of the diagnostic thresholds on the OGTT, but women who pass the OGTT, or who fail only one value, are at risk of delivering a macrosomic infant. Because of the higher incidence of macrosomia, women with one abnormal value on the OGTT warrant closer surveillance with either medical nutrition therapy and blood glucose monitoring or with a repeat OGTT 1 month later, when insulin resistance of pregnancy has increased further (Bevier, Fischer & Jovanovic, 1999).

Women who are having the GCT do not need to fast, but the nurse should advise them not to eat, drink, smoke or walk around during the test. Women who are scheduled for the OGTT should fast for at least 8 hours before the test, with at least 150 g of carbohydrate intake for 3 days preceding the test, and normal activity level. The nurse should also advise them not to eat, drink, smoke or walk around during the test.

Researchers have studied more economic and palatable methods for screening and diagnosing GDM. Lamar and colleagues (1999) administered 50 g of jelly beans, rather than 50 g of glucose drink, and found similar glucose responses with fewer side effects. However, small sample sizes consisting of women who were not at high risk for GDM may have affected results. Because solids and liquids vary in glycemic indices and differ in absorption rates, further research is needed to confirm the validity and safety of alternative testing for diabetes in pregnancy.

Researchers have also studied prediction of GDM by using the fasting plasma glucose (FPG). Atilano and colleagues (1999) found that an FPG of 105 mg/dL is significantly predictive of positive glucose results. The FPG has also been used to determine which women require the OGTT, thus omitting the GCT (Agarwal, Hughes, Punnose & Ezimokhai, 2000; Perucchini et al., 1999). These findings reduced the number of women who required the diagnostic OGTT. Further study with larger sample sizes, different risk categories and more diverse, representative populations are necessary before the current standard for GDM testing is replaced.

Metabolic Management During Pregnancy

Medical Nutrition Therapy

The goal of medical nutrition therapy during pregnancy is similar for women with pregestational and gestational diabetes—adequate nourishment and weight gain and prevention of ketosis and postprandial hyperglycemia. Women with type 1 and 2 diabetes need nutritional assessment as soon as pregnancy has been confirmed and ongoing evaluation throughout the pregnancy, making adjustments as indicated. Women with gestational diabetes require a nutritional assessment and plan as soon after diagnosis as possible. Figure 7 is a sample medical nutrition history and education checklist.

The medical nutritional therapy plan for the pregnant woman with diabetes should be individualized to her particular needs and lifestyle. As with the preconception MNT visit, pertinent data regarding the woman should be obtained before the visit (e.g., findings from the history and physical examination; laboratory test results; anthropometric data; medications; other health problems; physical activity and any restrictions; lifestyle factors including cultural, ethnic or religious influences; and complementary therapies) (Biastre, 2001). In addition, gastrointestinal issues, such as nausea and vomiting, eating disorders, food allergies or intolerances, cravings and aversions, should be explored (Biastre, 2001). A dietary recall or a diet diary should be obtained and evaluated in conjunction with blood glucose levels and insulin regimen. In women with

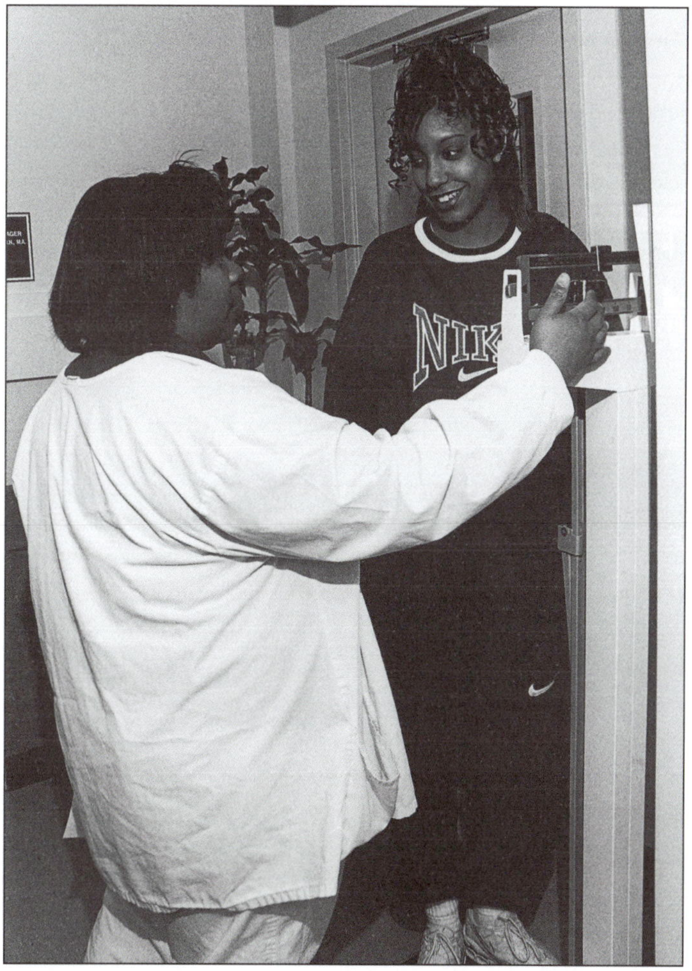

Figure 7. Medical Nutrition History and Education Checklist

Name____________________ Age__________ Date __________

Date of birth__________ Diabetes type__________ Age at diagnosis__________ Expected date of confinement __________

Gravida__________ Parity__________ Previous OB complications __________

Glucose challenge test & date__________ Oral glucose tolerance test & date__________ Fasting blood sugar______ 1 hr ____ 2 hr ____ 3 hr ____

Height______ Current weight_______ Pregravid weight________ % ideal/adjusted body weight________ Gestational age ________

Pregnancy weight gain__________ Insulin regimen __________

Medications __________

Past medical history __________

Occupation__________ Work hours __________

Referring provider __________

Expected Outcome	Date
Identifies rationale for the meal plan to achieve weight goal and normoglycemia	
Understands carbohydrate counting	
Uses methods to avoid hypoglycemia, including food spacing, portion size and food variety	
Understands abnormal blood glucose values based on changes in food intake (extra carbohydrate, skipped snacks, exercise, insulin or illness) and other variables, such as increasing pregnancy hormone levels	
Eliminates foods with a high glycemic index, such as regular sodas and concentrated sweets	
Uses blood glucose self-monitoring and food records to problem solve and/or identify blood glucose patterns related to food intake and the need for insulin or insulin adjustments	
Understands the role of exercise to improve blood glucose; adjusts diet to avoid hypoglycemia	
Understands appropriate use of artificial sweeteners and caffeine intake	
Reads food labels and understands grocery shopping guidelines	
Demonstrates knowledge of menu ideas and restaurant choices	
Understands sick day guidelines and hyperemesis	

Calories__________ (__________ meals and __________ snacks) % Carbohydrate__________ % Fat__________ % Protein__________

Return appointment/diet diary review__________

newly diagnosed gestational diabetes, nutritional counseling and blood glucose testing may occur simultaneously. A follow-up visit is needed after a few days or a week to evaluate food intake in relation to blood glucose results. Dietary manipulation may then occur, or initiation of insulin may be required if postprandial hyperglycemia cannot be blunted by diet alone.

Daily caloric intake should be based on the woman's weight and activity level and usually has to be increased by only 300 kcal/day (2nd and 3rd trimesters) to meet the increased energy requirements of pregnancy (Biastre, 2001). Women who are at desirable body weight require 30 kcal/kg/day to gain approximately 25 to 35 pounds (Jovanovic, 2000). Women who are at 120 percent to 150 percent ideal body weight require fewer calories (24 kcal/kg/day) to gain approximately 15 pounds. Underweight women who are <90 percent ideal body weight should consume 36 to 40 kcal/kg/day to gain 28 to 40 pounds. Overweight women who are >150 percent ideal body weight do not need to gain as much weight (15 pounds), but they should consume 12 to 18 kcal/kg/day (Jovanovic, 2000). These are general guidelines.

The focus of the diet should be on adequate nutrition, normoglycemia and avoidance of ketosis, not on weight gain alone. The distribution of calories should be 40 percent to 50 percent carbohydrate, 20 percent protein and 30 percent to 40 percent fat, with less than one-third of the fat calories from saturated fat, one-third from polyunsaturated fat and the balance from monounsaturated fats (Jovanovic, 2000). To supply continuous glucose and balance insulin, the woman can consume the carbohydrate content of the diet in three meals and three snacks. This may require adjustment to the woman's lifestyle, activity level and insulin requirements. Consistency in the carbohydrate content of food at meals and snacks is important to allow for insulin adjustments and to prevent excursions in the blood glucose. Ingestion of foods high in soluble fiber also helps prevent

Figure 8. Food Guide Pyramid Adapted for Pregnant Women

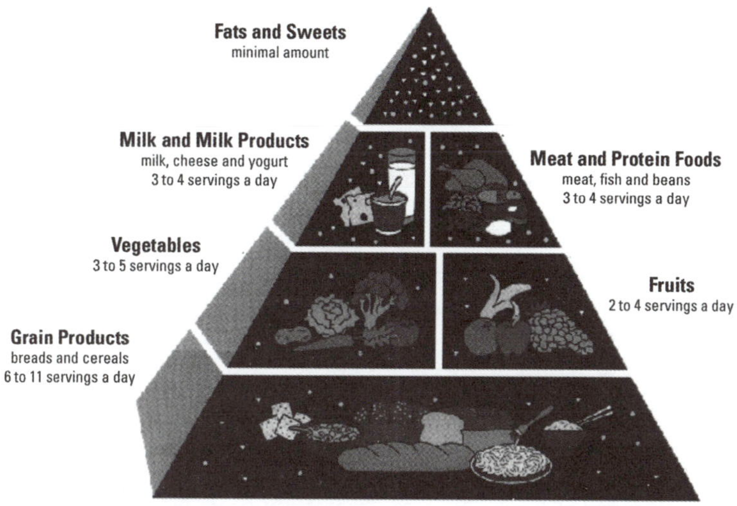

From March of Dimes, 2002

For pregnant women with diabetes, exercise may be beneficial for metabolic control and overall well-being when safety issues are addressed and precautions taken.

swings in the blood glucose by delaying absorption of glucose in the intestine (Jovanovic, 2000). The woman should avoid long periods of fasting to prevent starvation ketosis. A bedtime snack will usually offset early morning ketosis. Figure 8 provides the U.S. Department of Agriculture's Food Guide Pyramid adapted for pregnant women (March of Dimes, 2002).

The meal plan should include nutrients pertinent to pregnancy. Protein intake should be increased by 10 grams. The woman should consume 1,200 mg/day of calcium, 30 mg/day of iron (usually in a vitamin supplement) and 400 mcg/day of folate (Homko & Jornsay, 2001). Restriction of sodium is unnecessary. The woman should limit caffeine intake to 300 mg/day, which amounts to approximately 2 cups of coffee, to minimize the risk of intrauterine growth restriction associated with excessive caffeine intake (Jovanovic, 2000). The woman may safely use non-nutritive or artificial sweeteners (aspartame, saccharin, acesulfame potassium and sucralose) during pregnancy to reduce carbohydrate intake. Women with phenylketonuria should avoid aspartame.

Exercise

For pregnant women with diabetes, exercise may be beneficial for metabolic control and overall well-being when safety issues are addressed and precautions taken. Acute effects of exercise generally result in lowering of plasma glucose, with insulin sensitivity and glucose tolerance improvements occurring as a result of chronic exercise (Carpenter, 2000; Langer, 2000; Mulooly, 2001). The specific amount and type of exercise to promote lowering blood glucose has not been determined, although three episodes per week for at least 20 minutes seems to be required (Langer, 2000). Exercise has been shown to decrease the development of gestational diabetes in women at risk and also to obviate the need for insulin to control diabetes in women with GDM (Bung, Artal, Khodiguian & Kjos, 1991; Dye, Knox, Artal, Aubry & Wojtowycz, 1997).

Hypoglycemia is the most frequently encountered risk with exercise in individuals with diabetes, pregnant or nonpregnant. In individuals without diabetes, plasma insulin levels decrease during exercise, and counterregulatory hormones increase, allowing for hepatic glucose production and lipolysis to provide adequate glucose for utilization (Mulooly, 2001). In women with diabetes on insulin, the plasma insulin concentration does not decrease with exercise. However, insulin sensitivity may increase, and pools of insulin will mobilize, creating an increase in insulin levels that contributes to low blood glucose (BG) (Mulooly, 2001). Hepatic glucose production is inhibited in the face of higher plasma insulin concentrations. In addition, in individuals with impaired counterregulatory hormone response, hepatic glucose production is further inhibited and leads to hypoglycemia. Acute episodes of hypoglycemia may occur, but late onset hypoglycemia also may occur in women with type 1 diabetes as a result of increased insulin sensitivity and ongoing glucose utilization. Evaluation of blood glucose before, during and after exercise allows for appropriate insulin adjustments and determines the need for a reduction in insulin or an increase in carbohydrate supplementation. A reduction of rapid-acting insulin is recommended if exercise occurs during the peak action. If insulin is not reduced, additional carbohydrates will be required unless exercise occurs 1 to 3 hours after a meal. Before deciding to reduce insulin or increase carbohydrate supplementation, the woman should consider the time of exercise in relation to insulin and the previous meal, and the type, intensity and duration of exercise (Mulooly, 2001).

For women using an insulin pump, options to avoid hypoglycemia with exercise include suspending basal insulin during exercise, reducing basal insulin during exercise or increasing carbohydrate consumption (Mulooly, 2001). The ADA (2003f) recommends a graded exercise test before engaging in moderate- to high-intensity exercise for individuals who are older than 35; have had type 2 diabetes for longer than 10 years or type 1 diabetes for more than 15 years; are at risk for coronary artery disease; or have microvascular disease (proliferative retinopathy or nephropathy, including microalbuminuria), peripheral vascular disease or autonomic neuropathy. These recommendations also apply to pregnant women with diabetes. Table 14 lists ACOG's contraindications to exercise during pregnancy for women with or without diabetes.

Initiation of strenuous exercise during pregnancy is not recommended; however, most women can engage safely in walking, stationary cycling and swimming. Women who have already been involved in rigorous exercise, such as jogging or moderate- to high-intensity aerobics, should decrease sessions to 45 minutes and pay close attention to fatigue and other symptoms indicating stress to the pregnancy (Artal & Sherman, 1999). They should avoid lifting heavy weights; however, lifting light weights with moderate repetitions minimizes ligament and joint injury during pregnancy (Artal & Sherman, 1999). Periodic evaluation by the obstetric and diabetes provider is necessary to evaluate the effects of exercise on diabetes and the pregnancy. Table 15 identifies general precautions for women with diabetes who exercise.

Table 14. Contraindications to Exercise for Pregnant Women

- Pregnancy-induced hypertension
- Premature rupture of the membranes
- History of preterm labor
- Incompetent cervix/cerclage
- Persistent second and third trimester bleeding
- Intrauterine growth retardation

From ACOG, 1994

Self-Management

Comprehensive management of diabetes during pregnancy is vital to a successful outcome for both the woman and her infant. Self-management of diabetes in pregnancy includes self-monitoring of blood glucose, urine ketone testing and record keeping. Monitoring results provides the woman and her diabetes management team the information necessary to adjust the treatment plan.

Self-Monitoring of Blood Glucose

Self monitoring of blood glucose (SMBG) in pregnancy is the most important parameter for determining the level of metabolic control. A woman who monitors her own blood glucose can determine achievement of glycemic goals, the presence of hypoglycemia, the need for insulin or dietary adjustments, the effect of exercise or physical activity, the effect of food on glucose levels and the effect of stress and illness on blood glucose (Peragallo-Dittko, 2001). For women with gestational diabetes on MNT, SMBG determines the need for insulin.

Self monitoring of blood glucose (SMBG) in pregnancy is the most important parameter for determining the level of metabolic control.

A variety of blood glucose meters are available for home use. Meter selection should be based on a woman's needs or limitations (visual or hearing

Table 15. General Precautions for Women with Diabetes Who Exercise

- Wear proper, well-fitted footwear, including silica gel or air midsoles.
- Wear polyester or blend socks to maintain dryness.
- Inspect feet daily and after exercise.
- Avoid exercising in temperature extremes.
- Avoid exercising supine.
- Allow adequate warm-up and cooldown time (5 to 10 minutes for each).
- Monitor uterine activity; discontinue if present.
- Maintain adequate hydration.
- Avoid exercise during periods of poor metabolic control.
- Avoid exercising with blood glucose of 200 mg/dL with ketosis.
- Check blood glucose before exercising, after 30 minutes of exercise and 2 to 4 hours after exercise; consume carbohydrate supplement with BG of 100 mg/dL.
- Discontinue exercising if dizziness, shortness of breath, palpitations, excessive fatigue, pain or decreased fetal movement occurs.
- Have a carbohydrate snack available.
- Wear personal and diabetes identification.
- Exercise with others, if possible.
- Exercise at the same time each day; postprandial exercise decreases the risk of hypoglycemia.
- Consult your health care provider or diabetes educator to assist with insulin adjustments.

Adapted from ADA, 2003f; Artal & Sherman, 1999

impairment) and on reimbursement by a third-party payer. Two types of meters are used for SMBG. With color-reflectance meters, the blood drop reacts with an enzyme to produce a color change based on the amount of glucose in the blood (Peragallo-Dittko, 2001). Sensor meters measure the electronic charge generated by the chemical reaction between the enzyme and the glucose and provide a numeric result.

Neither meter is completely accurate. Accuracy is based on comparison to laboratory values and should be within 10 percent. The laboratory measures venous plasma blood glucose, whereas a meter measures a capillary sample of whole blood. The capillary sample, due to dilution, is approximately 11 percent to 15 percent lower than the plasma sample. Some meters calculate the plasma value based on whole blood and may be programmed to display whole blood or plasma values. Glycemic levels should be interpreted based on the level the meter reports, and glycemic goals should be given for whole blood and plasma. In addition, the level at which hypoglycemia is treated should be clarified based on plasma or whole blood. Table 16 provides ADA (2003d) recommendations for whole blood and plasma glycemic goals for pregnancy. Meter accuracy is also affected by user error, dehydration, hematocrit (low or high), altitude, improperly stored strips, environmental temperature extremes, humidity and some medications (Passanza, 2001).

The FDA has approved several meters that offer alternate site testing, in addition to fingerstick sampling, to minimize pain. If using the forearm as an alternate site, the individual must massage the forearm for at least 15 seconds before obtaining the sample. Because of the circulatory difference between the finger and forearm, failure to rub the forearm may result in a value that is much higher than a capillary sample obtained from the finger. This could pose a risk for individuals who use the forearm when they are experiencing hypoglycemia and do not take time to rub the arm before puncture (Jungheim & Koschinsky, 2001; McGarraugh, 2001). In a recent study, accuracy of samples from alternate sites was similar to fingerstick samples; most patients felt that alternate site testing was less painful and easy to perform (Fineberg, Bergenstal, Bernstein, Laffel & Schwartz, 2001). Regardless of the site used, patients should receive adequate instruction on the use of their glucose monitor and should understand the meter's limitations. The nurse should observe the woman's technique for obtaining a sample and ensure quality controls for the meter. Women testing for the first time will need thorough education and support for this aspect of diabetes management.

Timing and frequency of blood glucose testing are based on diabetes type and insulin regimen. Women with GDM should initially test fasting daily, 1 to 2 hours after each meal, while evaluating the effect of the diet on blood glucose and the need for insulin. After the effectiveness of the diet has been established, they can test less frequently. However, women should understand the importance of following the diet even when not testing. They should also know that, as pregnancy advances and concentrations of diabetogenic hormones increase, they may require insulin. Women with GDM who require insulin should test throughout pregnancy to allow for insulin adjustment. Women with type 1 and 2 diabetes should test fasting and 1 to 2 hours after meals, depending on whether they are using rapid- or immediate-acting insulin. Bedtime blood glucose testing is also important to help minimize nocturnal hypoglycemia. For women with hypoglycemia unawareness, a 2:00 a.m. to 3:00 a.m. blood glucose test is important to evaluate the effect of the intermediate acting insulin and allow adjustment to prevent nocturnal hypoglycemia. Women who take multiple daily injections of insulin or who use CSII need preprandial testing.

Urine Ketone Testing

Women should have daily urine ketone testing of the first voided specimen to rule out starvation ketosis, an indica-

Table 16. Glycemic Goals for Pregnancy

Timing	Whole Blood Glucose (mg/dL)	Plasma Glucose (mg/dL)
Fasting	<95	<105
Premeal	<105	<115
1 hour postprandial	<140	<155
2 hours postprandial	<120	<130

From ADA, 2003d

Successful self-administration of insulin requires patience, support and reassurance from the nurse educator to alleviate the woman's anxiety.

tion of inadequate food intake. Obese women with calorie-restricted diets should also perform daily urine ketone monitoring to detect insufficient caloric or carbohydrate intake (ADA, 2003d). The woman should test for urine ketones during periods of nausea and vomiting and when blood glucose levels are >200 mg/dL. Women should report moderate to large amounts of ketones to the health care provider immediately to allow for early intervention to prevent ketoacidosis.

Recordkeeping

Keeping records of blood glucose levels, urine ketone testing, dietary intake, timing and dosage of insulin and activity level allows for more appropriate adjustment of the diabetes regimen. Evaluating blood glucose levels alone does not provide all the information needed to fine tune the diabetes management plan. Meter data often can be downloaded into a computer, but this capability does not replace the value of a written log that designates meals and eating patterns. The nurse should periodically check meter memory to detect falsification and over- and under-reporting. When a lack of precision is detected, the nurse should explore causes with the woman and help her accept the need for more intensive management of diabetes during pregnancy.

To identify excursions in hyperglycemia undetected by postprandial self-monitoring, researchers compared the continuous glucose monitoring system (CGMS) to SMBG in a small sample of women with GDM. CGMS detected 4.7 episodes of hyperglycemia (>120 mg/dL), with 4.3 >130 mg/dL (Ilic, Jovanovic & Jeng, 2000). The authors found 2.4 episodes of undetected hypoglycemia of <60 mg/dL. They concluded that the risk of macrosomia in women with GDM who were thought to be in good glycemic control may be due to undetected and untreated hyperglycemia.

Insulin Therapy

Gestational Diabetes Mellitus

When medical nutrition therapy fails to achieve euglycemia in women with GDM, insulin is required. The dosage and timing of exogenous insulin is based on the pattern of hyperglycemia. Usually, two injections of a short and intermediate acting insulin are administered before breakfast and dinner. Dosage can be based on the woman's weight and gestational age, requiring 0.6 U/kg/day to 0.7 U/kg/day in the second trimester and 0.8 U/kg/day to 0.9 U/kg/day in the third trimester as contrainsulin hormones rise (Homko & Khandelwal, 1996). Women who are obese generally are more insulin resistant and require 1 U/kg/day to 2 U/kg/day to maintain metabolic control (Homko & Jornsay, 2001). Only human insulins are used during pregnancy because of their shorter duration of activity, more rapid onset and low level of immunogenicity.

The nurse should educate the woman and her family as soon as possible about all aspects of insulin administration. Successful self-administration of insulin requires patience, support and reassurance from the nurse educator to alleviate the woman's anxiety. The nurse should assure the woman that her need for insulin does not mean failure on her part. The nurse should individualize the education to the woman's learning needs. Table 17 identifies information to teach the woman about insulin administration.

Nurses should encourage women to use the abdomen for injection because this site allows the most rapid absorption of insulin, followed by the arms, thighs and buttocks. Women should rotate sites to improve consistency in

Table 17. Education Topics for Insulin Administration

- Glycemic goals for treatment, including the review of glucose log and the need for insulin
- Onset, peak and duration of insulin to be administered
- Insulin inspection, storage and travel precautions
- Site selection and regional rotation
- Technique for admixing insulin (single and mixed dose), self-administration and use of insulin pens
- Syringe and pen-needle disposal guidelines
- Signs and symptoms of hypoglycemia and appropriate treatment interventions
- Glucagon use for family and significant others
- Sick day management guidelines
- Indications for assessment of urine ketones
- When and how to call a health care provider

insulin absorption. They need to know how to identify and treat hypoglycemia and how to manage diabetes and insulin during periods of nausea and vomiting. Most women can self-inject insulin without difficulty and are surprised at the lack of discomfort and the ease of injection. Women who have difficulty with injection may consider using self-injector pens. If the woman cannot correctly draw up insulin, the nurse or a family member can prefill the insulin and store it in the refrigerator for up to 30 days. Insulin should be room temperature before injection to minimize discomfort. After the initial education session, the nurse should follow up within a week and be available by phone for questions or concerns. Because anti-insulin hormones increase throughout pregnancy, insulin adjustments are required every 1 to 2 weeks.

The FDA has not approved oral antidiabetes agents for use during pregnancy. However, a recent study showed that glyburide during the early second and third trimester controlled hyperglycemia as effectively as insulin in women with GDM, and it did not cross the placenta or result in adverse neonatal reactions (Langer, Conway, Berkus, Xenaki & Gonzales, 2000). Sulfonylureas have been found to cross the placenta with resultant neonatal hypoglycemia postulated to result from enhanced hyperinsulinemia in the infant (Kemball et al., 1970). Further study is warranted before these and similar drugs can be deemed safe for use during pregnancy.

Pregestational Diabetes Mellitus

Women with type 2 diabetes controlled by oral antidiabetes agents who become pregnant should discontinue these agents and begin insulin therapy. Education, counseling and follow-up should be the same as for women with gestational diabetes mellitus. Women with type 1 diabetes should review all aspects of insulin administration; the nurse should observe them drawing up and self-injecting insulin and provide appropriate education. Women with pregestational diabetes, particularly type 1 diabetes, are more prone to hypoglycemia and may also have hypoglycemia unawareness. Intensive management will result in hypoglycemia, and the nurse and woman should discuss prevention strategies and appropriate interventions. The nurse should review the increasing insulin requirements of pregnancy and advise the woman that the dosage at the end of pregnancy will be two to three times

The FDA has not approved oral antidiabetes agents for use during pregnancy.

higher than the prepregnancy dose (Jovanovic, 2000).

Continuous Subcutaneous Insulin Infusion

CSII, or insulin pump therapy, is another method of insulin delivery that has been used successfully in pregnancy. An insulin pump is an electronic device programmed to deliver a continuous low-dose infusion through a subcutaneously implanted catheter. Insulin boluses are delivered before meals and snacks, based on a predetermined insulin-to-carbohydrate intake ratio. Women who enter pregnancy already successfully using an insulin pump may continue to do so, but they will need education regarding the prevention of diabetic ketoacidosis (DKA), which develops more rapidly during the third trimester. Pump malfunction leaves the woman with no basal insulin, resulting in profound hyperglycemia. In pregnancy, conversion to fat metabolism with resultant ketone production will occur quickly, predisposing development of DKA. Pregnant women utilizing the pump should check their blood glucose frequently, self-inject for levels >200 mg/dL and troubleshoot the device. Some providers recommend using a low dose of intermediate-acting insulin at bedtime to reduce the risk of DKA development during the night, should an interruption in insulin delivery occur (Marcus & Fernandez, 1996). Another prudent approach is to check blood glucose levels at 2:00 a.m. or 3:00 a.m.

Initiation of CSII therapy during pregnancy requires careful patient selection. Candidates for CSII include women who are willing to test their blood glucose six to eight times daily and who can learn to program an electronic device. A woman may begin insulin pump therapy on an outpatient basis if she has adequate support and is in close contact with the diabetes provider. If concerns exist, hospitalization is a better option. Table 18 identifies initial insulin doses for pump therapy. During the first 48 hours after pump initiation, women should check their blood glucose fasting, premeals, 1-hour postprandial of meals and at bedtime, 12:00 midnight, 3:00 a.m. and 6:00 a.m. This allows adjustments of the basal rate based on multiple blood

Table 18. Initial Insulin Doses for Insulin Pump Therapy

Method 1 (Gabbe, 2000)

Calculate the initial insulin dose for the pump by the gestational age and weight of the woman as follows:

- First trimester—0.8 U/kg
- Second trimester—1.0 U/kg
- Third trimester—1.2 U/kg

Method 2 (Jornsay, 1998)

Calculate the initial insulin dose for the pump based on the total insulin dose as follows:

- Reduce the total daily insulin dose by 25 percent
- Administer 40 percent as an hourly basal rate
- Administer 60 percent as boluses with 25 percent at breakfast, 15 percent at lunch and 15 percent at dinner
- Use a lower basal rate during the night to minimize the risk of nocturnal hypoglycemia

glucose readings and more accurately reflects insulin needs. As pregnancy advances, adjustments will be required every 1 to 2 weeks. If the nighttime basal rate is increased, the woman should obtain a blood glucose at 2:00 a.m. or 3:00 a.m.

The ADA recommends Humalog, (lispro insulin) and Novolog (insulin aspart) as immediate acting insulin analogs, but they have not been approved by the FDA for use during pregnancy by injection or for pump therapy (ADA, 2003a). A study of lispro use during pregnancy did not find increased immunologic effects in women with gestational diabetes (Jovanovic et al., 1999). The authors also found fewer instances of hypoglycemia in the lispro-treated group. In a study of pregnant women with all diabetes types, the authors found only one difference between women using regular insulin and those using lispro: the hemoglobin A1C in the lispro group was lower before delivery (Bhattacharyya, Brown, Hughes & Vice, 2001). In a case report of three women treated with insulin lispro during pregnancy, diabetic retinopathy worsened to proliferative retinopathy (Kitzmiller, Main, Ward, Theiss & Peterson, 1999). The underlying cause of this finding was not known, but the authors theorized that strict improvement of glycemia may have been a contributing factor. Insulin lispro is a homolog of growth hormone IGF-1, which is currently under investigation in the development of diabetic retinopathy (Kitzmiller, Main, Ward, Theiss & Peterson, 1999). Randomized controlled studies need to be done to determine the safety and efficacy of lispro use during pregnancy.

Education and Counseling

As soon as pregnancy has been confirmed in women with pre-existing diabetes, they should receive comprehensive education and counseling. Women with gestational diabetes should receive education as soon as the diagnosis is made. All previous education should be reinforced, and the woman and her diabetes management team should set mutual goals. Figure 9 provides a documentation tool and guide for educating pregnant women with pregestational and gestational diabetes. Including family members and significant others in education sessions broadens the woman's support base.

Psychosocial Issues

Pregnant women with pre-existing diabetes display greater anxiety and hostility than pregnant women who do not have diabetes (Langer & Langer, 1998). This finding is not associated with the level of glycemic control. Women with more severe diabetes show lower compliance with follow-up visits, regardless of level of glycemic control (Langer & Langer, 1998). These and other emotional and psychosocial

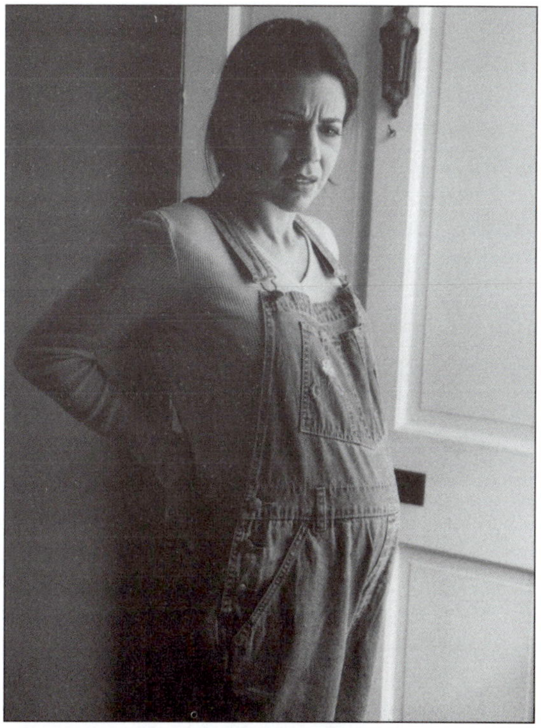

Figure 9. Diabetes in Pregnancy Education Checklist

Name______________________________ Date of birth____________ Age________

Diabetes type____________ Age @ diagnosis________ Expected date of confinement__________ Educator __________

Blood pressure________ Height_____ Weight_____ Urine: Protein_____ Glucose_____ Ketone_____

Glucose tolerance test: Fasting blood sugar____ 1h____ 2h____ 3h ____________________

The pregnant woman with diabetes will demonstrate the following:

Expected Outcome	Date
Understands diabetes, role of glucose and insulin transport	
Understands significance to pregnancy of 3-hour glucose tolerance test results (GDM)	
Understands effect pregnancy has on diabetes control, including role of placental hormones	
Understands potential outcomes of uncontrolled blood glucose—macrosomia, polyhydramnios, respiratory distress syndrome, preterm delivery, intrauterine fetal death, neonatal hypoglycemia, ketoacidosis, birth trauma, cesarean delivery	
Understands significance of Hemoglobin A1C for spontaneous abortion and congenital defects	
Uses glucose meter, including quality controls	
Uses autolancet to obtain blood sample with appropriate disposal	
Understands diabetes diet/diary and role of exercise, with safety guidelines	
Records technique of blood glucose values and abnormal reactions	
Understands glycemic goals for treatment	
Knows onset and peak times of prescribed insulin	
Inspects and stores insulin correctly	
Draws up insulin correctly (single and mixed)	
Identifies timing of injection, injection sites, rotation and technique and appropriate syringe disposal	
Identifies signs and symptoms of hypoglycemia	
Treats hypoglycemia with documented low (written guidelines)	
Has support person with knowledge of glucagon use and appropriate administration—provided Rx with two refills	
Identifies signs and symptoms of ketoacidosis; reports persistent nausea/vomiting, illness, infection, persistent hyperglycemia or recurrent insulin reactions	
Checks ketones daily with first void (pregestational) and with blood glucose values >180 mg/dL	
Understands sick day management (written guidelines)	
Schedules antepartum testing	
Understands significance of GDM for future pregnancy, development of overt DM later in life, appropriate follow-up, need for follow-up testing, preconception control and risk-minimizing interventions	
Understands significance of diabetes and development of long-term complications related to poor control	

Level of comprehension__________________ Learning impediments __________________

Family support____________ Previous education____________ Meter ____________

Adapted from Kendrick, 1999

issues need to be explored. Although the woman enters pregnancy with coping mechanisms in place to deal with her diabetes, the additional demands and concerns of pregnancy complicate the disorder. She may have experienced a previous loss from miscarriage or fetal death and have unresolved grief or heightened anxiety regarding the outcome of this pregnancy. The diabetes management team must support the woman and not judge or criticize. The team should not add to the woman's anxiety and hostility but, instead, should become her partner in dealing with all aspects of diabetes and pregnancy management. Not all women will be able to adhere to the ideal diabetes regimen for pregnancy. Mutually agreed upon goals for glycemia and self-monitoring are more valuable than those arbitrarily given to the woman without her input or without evaluation of her lifestyle. A psychosocial assessment is a vital component of diabetes management in pregnancy. Referrals should be made for findings that require mental health care intervention.

The woman's age affects diabetes management and psychosocial evaluation. Adolescents with diabetes have the same risk of pregnancy as those who do not have medical disorders. Nurses should be knowledgeable about adolescence, as well as about diabetes and pregnancy. Table 19 identifies the effects of diabetes on adolescent development. Adolescent females should be evaluated for eating disorders, which are more common in young girls with diabetes because diabetes requires a focus on food and eating (Betschart, 2001). Because weight gain is easily controlled by not taking insulin as prescribed, monitoring weight gain and ketosis is critical. An atmosphere of acceptance and support without criticism and judgment helps the teen accept the necessary diabetes regimen. The March of Dimes nursing module *Adolescent Pregnancy* (Breedlove & Schorfheide, 2001) offers a comprehensive guide for dealing with teen pregnancy.

Table 19. Effects of Diabetes on Adolescent Development

- Problems with self-image and identity (being identified as a diabetic)
- Difficulty achieving independence due to parental protectiveness or failure to accept responsibility of diabetes management
- Concerns about physical growth and development
- Attitudes of experimentation and rebellion, including risk behaviors regarding safe diabetes management

From Betschart, 2001

Because women with newly diagnosed gestational diabetes have a medical disorder that is likely to be temporary, they do not have the same stressors as do women who have preexisting diabetes. One study found that women with gestational diabetes have lower levels of depression and better glycemic control than do women with pregestational diabetes (Langer & Langer, 2000). In addition, women with GDM on intensified regimens that include insulin are no more anxious than women who are not on insulin. The goal of education for women with GDM is to empower them to be able to achieve metabolic control. Women who attain normoglycemia have a lower incidence of anxiety, fatigue, hostility and lack of confidence (Langer & Langer, 2000). The March of Dimes nursing module *Pregnancy: Psychosocial Perspectives*, 3rd Edition (Ramer & Frank, 2001) offers a comprehensive review of psychosocial issues related to pregnancy.

The goal of education for women with GDM is to empower them to be able to achieve metabolic control.

Women with gestational diabetes are at no greater risk than women without diabetes to deliver preterm, unless they have other complications that put them at risk.

Management of Acute Complications during Pregnancy

Preterm Labor

Women with gestational diabetes are at no greater risk than women without diabetes to deliver preterm, unless they have other complications that put them at risk. Women with pregestational diabetes with vascular disease or hypertensive disorders of pregnancy are at higher risk for preterm labor and birth. Nursing management of women with diabetes who are experiencing preterm labor requires skilled assessment and intervention to prevent complications from treatment. Preterm contractions may abate with fluids administered orally or intravenously (when oral fluids are not tolerated). Fluids containing glucose should be avoided unless the blood glucose level is <100 mg/dL. Bedside capillary blood glucose monitoring should be performed hourly and intravenous fluids titrated to maintain levels <120 mg/dL. Normal saline or regular insulin should be administered intravenously or subcutaneously if the blood glucose is >120 mg/dL.

The most commonly used medications to treat preterm labor are beta adrenergic agonists. These drugs should be used cautiously in women with diabetes because their use has been associated with hyperglycemia and hypokalemia. When oral beta adrenergic agonists are given to women with gestational diabetes who are diet-controlled, hyperglycemia thresholds may be exceeded and insulin will be required as long as preterm labor is treated. When beta adrenergic agonists are administered to treat preterm labor in women with insulin-controlled gestational diabetes or with pregestational diabetes, the insulin dose usually needs to be increased. Magnesium sulfate is safer than beta adrenergic agonists for women with diabetes because it does not result in hyperglycemia or hypokalemia; however, it must be administered intravenously and carries a risk of respiratory depression.

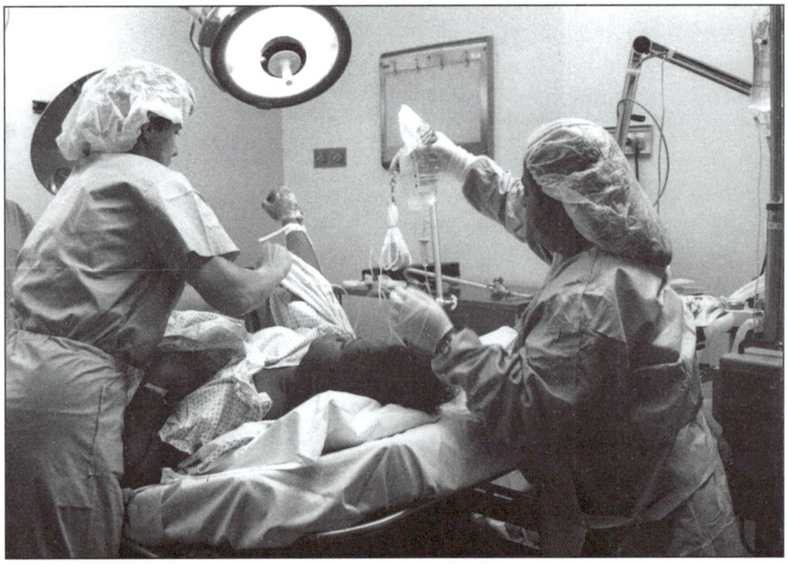

Corticosteroids are often given to accelerate fetal lung maturation in gestations <34 weeks expected to deliver within 1 week (Jovanovic, 2000). If administration of steroids results in hyperglycemia, close metabolic surveillance should be employed and the insulin dose adjusted to maintain euglycemia.

Hypoglycemia

Intensive metabolic management during pregnancy is associated with an increased incidence of hypoglycemia that has been reported as high as 71 percent, occurring primarily during the first and early second trimesters (Rosenn, Miodovnik, Holcberg, Khoury & Siddiqi, 1995). Rosenn and colleagues (1995) found that 34 percent of women with pre-existing diabetes had at least one episode of severe hypoglycemia that resulted in seizures, loss of consciousness, injury, glucagon administration and intravenous glucose therapy. Nausea and vomiting in early pregnancy, fetal siphoning of glucose and intensive insulin therapy contribute to the higher incidence of hypoglycemia in pregnancy. A decrease in counter-regulatory hormonal response to hypoglycemia during pregnancy has also been demonstrated (Bjorklund et al., 1998; Rosenn, Miodovnik, Khoury & Siddiqi, 1996). Studies of rat and mice embryos found associations of fetal malformations after short- and long-term hypoglycemia, but no studies have shown adverse outcomes in human fetuses. Contrarily, Bjorklund and colleagues (1998) found increased fetal movement and reactivity with normal umbilical artery flow velocity wave forms during moderate, insulin-induced hypoglycemia. Hypoglycemia, even if not teratogenic, can result in serious consequences in the woman. Neurocognitive functioning may be irreparably impaired with frequent episodes of severe hypoglycemia (Langan, Dreary, Hepburn & Frier, 1991).

Recurring episodes of hypoglycemia require further exploration to determine the underlying cause. Reviewing a food intake log, timing of insulin, level of activity or exercise and amount and timing of meals and snacks may reveal a pattern that contributes to the development of hypoglycemia that can easily be corrected. Frequent insulin adjustments, irregular timing of dosages and decreasing food intake without decreasing the insulin dose predisposes the woman to hypoglycemia. In addition, irregular timing of meals in relation to insulin, skipping meals and snacks or altering the content of the carbohydrate intake at a meal without making an insulin adjustment contributes to the development of hypoglycemia (Gonder-Frederick, 2001). Hypoglycemia may also result from increasing physical activity without adding carbohydrates or varying the daily activity schedule. Scheduling adjustments alone can minimize the risk of hypoglycemia. Episodes of nocturnal hypoglycemia are especially dangerous because the woman may not awaken to early symptoms. Checking blood glucose levels between 2:00 a.m. and 3:00 a.m., eating a snack before going to sleep and taking intermediate-acting insulin at bedtime decrease this risk.

Education for women and their significant others should include verbal and written information about recognition and treatment of hypoglycemia. Table 20 identifies hypoglycemia treatment instructions. Cognitive functioning after an episode of severe hypoglycemia varies and may take as long as 90 minutes to recover. Overtreatment of hypoglycemia is discouraged due to rebound hyperglycemia. Some women with diabetes may benefit from commercially prepared glucose products.

Table 20. Hypoglycemia Treatment

- Ingest 10 g to 15 g of carbohydrate, in liquid or solid form, for a blood glucose of 60 mg/dL, or 70 mg/dL for a plasma meter, to raise the blood glucose by 30 mg/dL to 45 mg/dL in 30 minutes (Gonder-Frederick, 2001).
- Do not consume foods high in fat and protein because they delay absorption.
- Ingest 20 g to 30 g of carbohydrate for blood glucose levels <50 mg/dL.
- Check the blood glucose every 15 minutes until the hypoglycemia is resolved.
- Eat food within 1 hour after a hypoglycemic episode to restore glycemic stores and to prevent a recurrence of hypoglycemia.
- Keep your meter and a carbohydrate source available at all times.

The incidence of DKA in pregnancy has decreased dramatically due to intensive glycemic control of diabetes in pregnancy and more comprehensive patient education emphasizing prevention strategies.

Diabetic Ketoacidosis

Diabetic ketoacidosis (DKA) is a rare occurrence in pregnancy, affecting only 1 percent to 3 percent of women with diabetes (Ramin, 1999). DKA is more likely to occur in women with type 1 diabetes but has been reported in women with type 2 and gestational diabetes. The incidence of DKA in pregnancy has decreased dramatically due to intensive glycemic control of diabetes in pregnancy and more comprehensive patient education emphasizing prevention strategies. However, devastating outcomes may result for the mother and fetus. Mortality rate for the mother is 5 percent in experienced centers (ADA, 2003e). Fetal loss is higher. Spontaneous abortion may result if DKA occurs in the first or early second trimester, with intrauterine fetal death occurring in late second or third trimester. Fetal loss has decreased to approximately 9 percent in the past decade due to improved perinatal management (Cullen, Reece, Homko & Sivan, 1996). Fetal mortality becomes significantly different in women with poorly controlled diabetes. Fetal loss in women with poor metabolic control has been reported as high as 48 percent with DKA, compared to 10 percent in women who had better glycemic control (Kent, Gill & Williams, 1994).

DKA occurs as a result of profound insulin deficiency. Small amounts of insulin may be circulating, but, due to the antagonistic action of stress hormones (glucagon, catecholamines, cortisol and growth hormone), the insulin is ineffective (Davidson, 2001). During the fed state, insulin deficiency results in impaired uptake of glucose in the peripheral tissues. During fasting, insulin deficiency leads to hyperglycemia by increasing hepatic glucose production (Davidson, 2001). Protein degradation as an energy source increases gluconeogenic amino acids, which increase hepatic glucose production, resulting in hyperglycemia. In the presence of high counterregulatory hormones, hydrolysis of stored fat occurs, releasing free fatty acids (FFAs) and glycerol. Glycerol is a gluconeogenic precurser that further increases liver production of glucose, increasing hyperglycemia. The liver converts FFAs to ketone bodies, leading to ketonemia and, eventually, to acidosis as the buffering capacity of the body is exceeded (Davidson, 2001). This process occurs more rapidly in pregnancy because of metabolic changes that result in a rapid conversion to fat metabolism during fasting and insulin deficient states.

Table 21 lists contributing clinical variables, signs and symptoms and diagnostic laboratory values associated with the development of DKA. Prevention of DKA in pregnancy focuses on education. Pregnant women with diabetes should daily test their urine from the first void for ketones to detect starvation ketosis. Inadequate food intake is usually the cause of early morning ketonuria when blood glucose levels are normal to low. A bedtime snack usually corrects early morning ketosis. Ketones present with elevated blood glucose levels may be an early indication of developing ketoacidosis. Ketones should also be checked with blood glucose levels of 180 mg/dL or greater because DKA can develop at much lower blood glucose levels in pregnancy. A thorough knowledge of insulin and dietary management during periods of nausea and vomiting should be evaluated. Pregnant women with diabetes should know to call their provider when they have nausea and vomiting with moderate to large amounts of ketonuria or when they are unable to lower their blood glucose with additional insulin.

As soon as pregnancy is confirmed, the woman should receive a prescription for anti-emetics to control vomiting. Because infection may lead to the development of DKA, the woman should be alert to signs and symptoms and report them to her provider, particularly in the presence of difficult to control blood glucose levels or ketonuria. Infection increases the release of insulin-antagonizing hormones, cortisol and catecholamines, resulting in hyperglycemia that is difficult to decrease with correction dosages of insulin.

Table 21 also identifies DKA laboratory confirmation. In addition to diagnostic tests, other laboratory tests are necessary to monitor the progress of treatment. These include a complete blood count (CBC), electrolytes, blood urea nitrogen (BUN), serum phosphorus, magnesium, ketones and a urinalysis with a culture and sensitivity (Davidson, 2001). An elevated leukocyte count does not provide the best indication of infection in DKA because of falsely elevated levels as a result of dehydration. An elevated band neutrophil count is a better indicator of infection. Serum ketones are necessary for diagnostic purposes but not for monitoring response to therapy. Serum ketones only measure one ketone body (acetoacetate) responsible for the development of DKA. The other ketone body that is present in equal amounts to acetoacetate is beta-hydroxybutyrate. As DKA resolves, beta-hydroxybutyrate converts back to acetoacetate, so serum ketones lag behind clinical improvement and may be present for days.

Table 21. Diabetic Ketoacidosis in Pregnancy

Contributing Clinical Factors
- Stress
- Emesis
- Infection
- Steroid administration
- Beta adrenergic agonists
- Insulin pump failure
- Noncompliance

Signs and Symptoms
- Abdominal pain
- Nausea and vomiting
- Polyuria
- Polydipsia
- Fruity breath
- Kussmaul respirations
- Leg cramps
- Altered mental status
- Hypotension
- Hypothermia

Laboratory Diagnostic Values (ADA, 2003e)
- Blood glucose >250 mg/dL
- Bicarbonate <15 mEq/L
- pH<7.3
- Moderate ketonuria

Immediate goals of DKA treatment are correction of the fluid deficit and electrolyte imbalance, reduction of hyperglycemia and detection and treatment of infection. Skilled and aggressive nursing and medical management of DKA in pregnancy is required to decrease maternal and fetal risk. Nurses who have combined obstetric and intensive care knowledge can render the most appropriate care. When a pregnant woman presents with DKA in a community hospital, she should be stabilized and transported to a tertiary care facility with high-risk perinatal services.

DKA may be classified as mild, moderate or severe based on patient presentation and laboratory values (ADA, 2003e). Mild DKA is characterized by a blood glucose >250 mg/dL, a pH of 7.35 to 7.30, a bicarbonate level of 15 to 18 with positive urine and serum

Skilled and aggressive nursing and medical management of DKA in pregnancy is required to decrease maternal and fetal risk. Nurses who have combined obstetric and intensive care knowledge can render the most appropriate care.

ketones in an alert patient (ADA, 2003e). Treatment for mild DKA consists of oral hydration of three to five ounces per hour if nausea and vomiting are not present (Davidson, 2001). Sugar-free beverages are recommended, but beverages containing sugar have been used successfully because, at this point, hydration is more important than blood glucose. Insulin should be supplemented by administering 10 percent to 20 percent of the usual total daily dose. Moderate DKA is diagnosed by hyperglycemia >250 mg/dL, a pH of 7.0 to 7.24, with a bicarbonate between 10 to 15 with positive urine and serum ketones in a drowsy patient (ADA, 2003e). Women with moderate to severe DKA cannot tolerate oral rehydration and require emergent care.

Table 22. Nursing Management of Diabetic Ketoacidosis in Pregnancy

Treatment	Nursing Intervention
Fluid resuscitation	1. Obtain large bore peripheral access. 2. Anticipate need for hemodynamic monitoring. 3. Administer fluids as ordered, usually 1,000 ml to 2,000 ml normal saline over 1 to 2 hours, then 200 ml/hour to 250 ml/hour. 4. Assess for signs and symptoms of pulmonary edema—dyspnea, tachypnea, wheezing, cough a. Assess for hypovolemia—Check vital signs every 15 minutes. Report decrease in blood pressure, increased pulse rate, decrease in central venous and pulmonary capillary wedge pressure and slow capillary refill. b. Insert Foley catheter if oliguria or anuria present. Send specimen for urinalysis, culture and sensitivity. c. Record hourly intake and output. Report output <30 ml/hour. d. Give 5 percent dextrose solution at blood glucose of 200 mg/dL to 250 mg/dL to prevent hypoglycemia.
Insulin therapy	1. Administer intravenous insulin as ordered—10 U to 20 U regular insulin bolus, then 5 U/hour to 10 U/hour. 2. Determine hourly capillary blood glucose (laboratory correlation with each blood draw). 3. Double dosage as ordered if 10 percent decrease in blood glucose is not achieved in the first hour. 4. Notify physician when blood glucose of 200 mg/dL is reached, anticipating decrease in insulin infusion rate to 1 U/hour to 2 U/hour. 5. Monitor for hypoglycemia. 6. Monitor for cerebral edema—headache, vomiting, deteriorating mental status, bradycardia, sluggish pupillary light reflex, widened pulse pressure.

(Continued on next page)

Table 22. Nursing Management of Diabetic Ketoacidosis in Pregnancy (cont'd.)

Treatment	Nursing Intervention
Electrolyte replacement	1. Apply ECG and report ST segment depression, inverted T waves and appearance of U waves after T waves. 2. Obtain hourly laboratory electrolyte levels. 3. Anticipate potassium replacement within 4 hours.
Oxygenation	1. Establish airway. 2. Anticipate placement of peripheral arterial catheter. 3. Obtain initial arterial blood gases, then hourly until pH of 7.20 is maintained. 4. Administer oxygen at 8 to 10 L/min via non-rebreathing face mask to maintain oxygen saturations of 95 percent. 5. Anticipate need for intubation/mechanical ventilation. 6. Continue pulse oximetry. 7. Administer bicarbonate as ordered for pH of 7.10.
Fetal/Uterine monitoring	1. Use the left lateral recumbent position. 2. Apply external fetal/uterine monitoring (EFM). 3. Observe EFM for evidence of fetal compromise. 4. Observe for uterine activity. 5. Administer tocolytics as ordered (MgSO4, drug of choice). 6. Avoid beta adrenergic agonists and steroids.

Fluid Resuscitation

Table 22 identifies nursing strategies and treatment modalities for the pregnant woman in DKA. Initial treatment focuses on correction of dehydration, which improves tissue perfusion and peripheral insulin delivery and decreases hyperglycemia by hemodilution (Davidson, 2001). Normal (0.9 percent) saline is the initial fluid of choice for rapid intravenous administration if the blood pressure is normal or low and serum sodium is <140 mg/dL. If the serum sodium is >155 mg/dL and the serum osmolality is >320 mosm/kg with a normal blood pressure, isotonic saline should be avoided and half-normal (0.45 percent) saline should be administered (Davidson, 2001). When the serum glucose falls to 200 mg/dL to 250 mg/dL, fluid administration should be changed to 5 percent dextrose to prevent the development of hypoglycemia and cerebral edema (Ramin, 1999).

Insulin Therapy

Intravenous regular insulin should be admixed and administered immediately per institution protocol or by physician's order via a controlled infusion device in a separate or piggybacked line after an initial bolus. Blood glucose will fall at a rate of 75 mg/dL to 100 mg/dL per hour with adequate hydration and insulin therapy (Davidson, 2001). After hyperglycemia has improved, intravenous insulin should be titrated according to blood glucose values for 12 to 24 hours to prevent a recurrence of DKA. Approximately 30 minutes to 1 hour before discontinuing intravenous insulin, subcutaneous insulin should be administered (Whiteman, Homko & Reece, 1996).

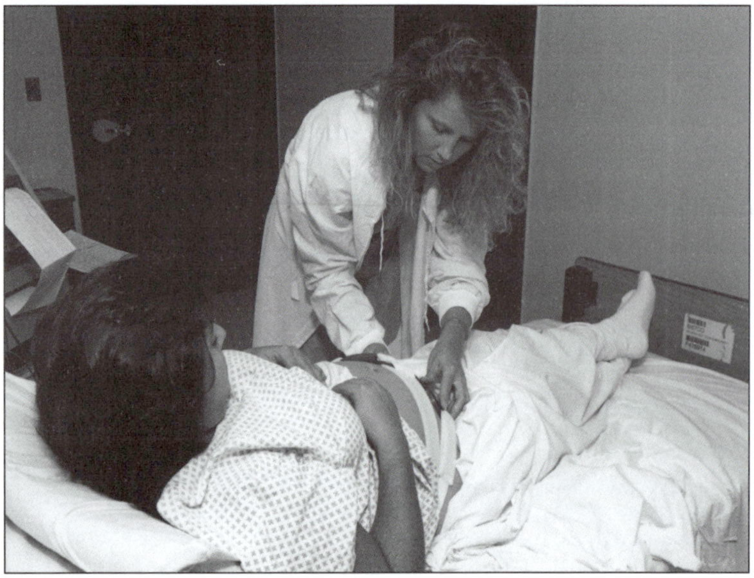

Electrolyte Replacement
The serum potassium level may be normal or elevated on admission due to dehydration and intracellular shift of potassium into the serum (Davidson, 2001). As long as there is adequate urinary output, potassium should be replaced as the acidosis resolves and intravascular volume is restored. The nurse should observe continuous ECG monitoring for indication of hypokalemia, evidenced by low or flattened T waves or U waves, in addition to serum monitoring of potassium levels. The ECG trace indicates hyperkalemia when peaked T waves or a widened QRS interval are present (Davidson, 2001). Bicarbonate administration is not usually indicated unless the pH is <7.1 when there is a risk of cardiac arrythmias. Replacement of bicarbonate at a pH level of 7.0 to 7.1 may result in too rapid a correction of the pH and pCO2, and may increase pCO2 in the fetus, further reducing oxygen delivery to maternal tissues (Ramin, 1999).

Fetal and Uterine Monitoring
The exact effect of maternal diabetic ketoacidosis on the fetus is unknown. It has been theorized that maternal metabolic acidosis and severe dehydration decrease uterine blood flow and result in fetal oxygen deprivation (Ramin, 1999). In addition, the metabolic disturbances in the mother are assumed to be duplicated in the fetus, because ketoacids and glucose readily cross the placenta (Whiteman, Homko & Reece, 1996). Fetal heart rate monitoring during DKA usually reveals a fetus in distress by the appearance of late decelerations, decreased beat-to-beat variability, non-reactive pattern or a non-reassuring biophysical profile (Chauhan & Perry, 1995). Cesarean intervention may result in further maternal deterioration without fetal benefit (Chauhan & Perry, 1995). To improve uterine perfusion, intrauterine resuscitative measures, such as maternal rehydration, left lateral recumbent position and adequate oxygenation, should be instituted. Maternal oxygenation status should be continually monitored by arterial blood gas determinations and continuous pulse oximetry. Oxygen saturations should be maintained at ≥95 percent or greater.

The pregnant woman in DKA may present with preterm uterine activity. Intervention should be individualized to the maternal status, gestational age and fetal condition (Chauhan & Perry, 1995). Uterine activity may subside with the mother's rehydration. If contractions persist coupled with cervical change, tocolytic therapy is indicated. The use of beta adrenergic agonists are contraindicated because of an associated risk of hyperglycemia, increase in free fatty acids and ketone production, which may escalate the hyperglycemic crisis (Chauhan & Perry, 1995). Magnesium sulfate is the tocolytic deemed safe for use during ketoacidosis. Administration of corticosteroids for fetal lung maturation should also be avoided due to associated hyperglycemia.

Psychosocial Issues
After resolution of DKA, the nurse should explore causes and prevention strategies with the woman and her family. The nurse should avoid criticism and educate the woman about early detection measures to allow for prompt intervention. Nurses can offer emotional support, reassurance and education. While DKA is treated, women may be anxious about their unborn infant and need continual information regarding fetal status. Women who deliver a premature infant as a result of DKA need special support from neonatal staff and should visit their infants as soon as they are stable. Pictures or videos of the infant may reassure an anxious mother. Some hospitals have closed-circuit videos for mothers who are unable to visit their infants in intensive care.

Women who experience fetal loss with DKA will need intensive support and grief counseling. Many hospitals have grief counselors to meet the needs of women who lose an infant. Feelings of guilt should be explored with the woman. Many women blame themselves, even when little could have been done to prevent the development of DKA. Follow-up to evaluate the woman's physical and psychological status should occur soon after discharge from the hospital. The March of Dimes offers a bereavement kit, available in English and Spanish, for families who have experienced loss (March of Dimes, 1999). Grieving during the perinatal period is also the focus of the March of Dimes nursing module *Loss and Grieving in Pregnancy and the First Year of Life: A Caring Resource for Nurses* (Gemma & Arnold, 2002).

Antepartum Maternal Surveillance
For women with pre-existing diabetes, a comprehensive antepartum assessment includes a history, physical examination and laboratory evaluation at the first prenatal visit. For women who are poorly controlled and in the period of organogenesis, this assessment should occur in the hospital for intensive metabolic management. In the following weeks, visit frequency should be based on the level of glycemic control and the presence of vascular disease. Women who require frequent insulin adjustments should be seen weekly or twice weekly. Women who have achieved a higher level of metabolic control may be seen biweekly. At each prenatal visit, the nurse should take vital signs, test urine for protein, glucose and ketones; review the self-management log; inspect injection sites for bruising, infection, lipohypertrophy or atrophy; and check the woman's weight. Weight gain that is not in the normal range requires further exploration with the dietician. Periodically, meter data should be downloaded and compared to logged values to ascertain accuracy. Hemoglobin A1C measurements should be taken every 4 to 6 weeks.

Pregnant women who have vascular disease require closer monitoring. Women with nephropathy require a 24-hour urine for protein and creatinine clearance and electrolyte assessment at a minimum of each trimester. Coagulation studies, uric acid and liver function should be obtained in each trimester. Visits should occur at least every 1 to 2 weeks in the first and second trimesters, and weekly to twice weekly in the third trimester, to closely evaluate blood pressure, urinary protein and edema. Hospitalization may be required in the third trimester for intensive surveillance if nephrotic syndrome develops. Women with a history of retinopathy need ophthalmologic evaluation each trimester.

Women with gestational diabetes mellitus, if diagnosed in the first trimester,

For women with pre-existing diabetes, a comprehensive antepartum assessment includes a history, physical examination and laboratory evaluation at the first prenatal visit.

The goals of antepartum fetal testing include elimination of stillbirth by early intervention, detection of fetal compromise, and prevention of unnecessary preterm delivery.

should be monitored in a similar fashion as women with pre-existing diabetes. Because 2 percent of women of reproductive age have undiagnosed type 2 diabetes mellitus, a physical examination and laboratory evaluation can rule out the presence of vascular disease (Homko & Jornsay, 2001). In addition, women diagnosed with GDM in the first trimester have been found to develop hypertension more frequently and have higher glycemic values that require insulin (Bartha, Martinez-Del-Fresno & Comino-Delgada, 2000). Women diagnosed with gestational diabetes between 24 to 28 weeks require weekly visits to evaluate the level of glycemic control. More frequent visits may be required for women who initiate insulin. Weight gain or loss should be monitored closely and evaluated by the dietician. As with women with pregestational diabetes, evaluation at prenatal visits should include assessment of vital signs, urine protein, ketones and glucose; inspection of injection sites for women self-administering insulin; and review of the self-management log. In addition to physical assessment, women with diabetes should be evaluated for tolerance of the diabetes regimen, including assessment for symptoms of depression and anxiety. Missing appointments may be an indication of depression.

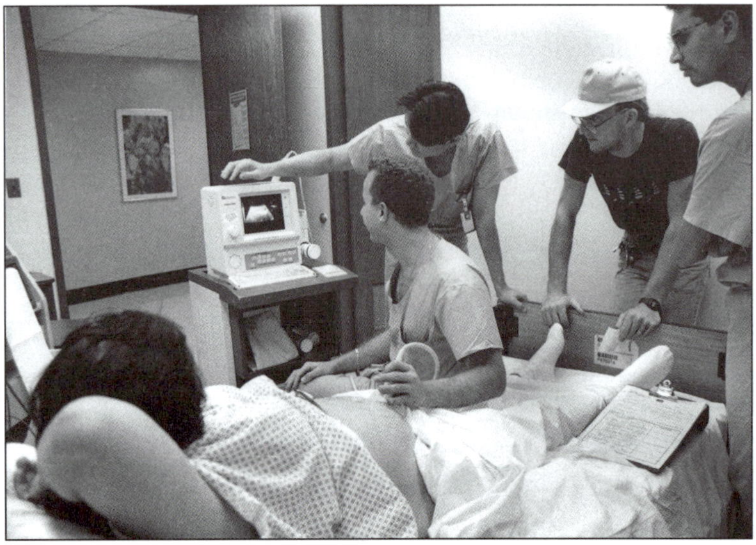

Antepartum Fetal Surveillance

Antepartum fetal surveillance is a standard of care for management of pregnancy complicated by diabetes. However, the best method and the appropriate time to begin fetal testing in diabetic pregnancy has yet to be determined. Table 23 provides a sample schedule for monitoring the fetus. The timing and type of antepartum fetal testing should take into consideration the woman's level of metabolic control, her obstetric history and the presence of vascular complications. The goals of antepartum fetal testing include elimination of stillbirth by early intervention, detection of fetal compromise, and prevention of unnecessary preterm delivery (Landon, 2000).

Pregnant women with pregestational diabetes should have fetal ultrasonography as early as possible to determine the period of organogenesis, the need for hospitalization for strict glycemic control and the anticipated delivery date. Early dating ultrasonography is important for women diagnosed with gestational diabetes in the first or early second trimester. Fetal nuchal translucent measurements may be obtained between 11 to 14 weeks. The ultrasound should be repeated between 20 to 22 weeks gestation to assess for fetal malformations. Women with poorly controlled diabetes or with vascular disease should receive fetal echocardiography to rule out fetal cardiac defects. Serial ultrasounds should be obtained beginning in the third trimester to assess fetal growth aberrations of macrosomia or intrauterine growth restriction (IUGR). Amniotic fluid volume should also be assessed for polyhydramnios, which may indicate poor maternal glycemic control, leading to fetal hyperglycemia and polyuria. Oligohydramnios is a more serious ultrasound finding and may occur in pregnancies complicated by vascular disease and hypertension.

Maternal serum alpha-fetoprotein (MSAFP) testing is recommended between 16 to 19 weeks gestation as an option to screen for neural tube defects, which occur at a much higher incidence in infants of mothers with diabetes. Women with type 1 diabetes have lower levels of MSAFP as compared to women without diabetes at each gestational age (Jovanovic, 2000). Chromosomal abnormality detection improves when multiple marker testing or triple screening is used. These tests measure human chorionic gonadotropin and estriol, in addition to MSAFP. An amniocentesis may be offered based on risks identified by these screening tests.

All pregnant women with gestational or pregestational diabetes should begin fetal movement counting or scoring in the third trimester (26 to 28 weeks gestation). Pregnant women should count movements after meals for a specified time period once or twice daily. A decrease in the specified frequency or intensity of perceived fetal movement warrants further testing.

Most centers use the nonstress test (NST) after 26 to 28 weeks gestation to evaluate the fetus in high-risk pregnancies complicated by diabetes. The NST involves placing two transducers from an external fetal monitor (EFM) on the maternal abdomen. One transducer records the fetal heart rate, and the other monitors uterine activity. The test is considered reactive or favorable if the fetal heart rate increases with activity or stimulation. A non-reactive pattern may indicate fetal compromise and requires further testing, usually with a biophysical profile (BPP) or a contraction stress test (CST). Table 23 includes a schedule for initiation of non-stress testing.

A CST involves the use of the external fetal monitor to evaluate fetal response to the stress of induced uterine contractions. Contractions are induced by administration of low-dose oxytocin to the mother or by maternal nipple stimulation. The EFM strip is observed for the presence of late decelerations that occur after 50 percent of the uterine contractions (Homko & Jornsay, 2001). The CST carries a small risk of preterm labor.

The BPP is used as a primary testing tool or when the NST is non-reactive. The BPP combines an ultrasound with the NST and evaluates four biophysical parameters: fetal breathing motion, gross body movements, fetal tone and amniotic fluid volume (Landon, 2000). The NST and each parameter receive a score of 2 if present (or reactive) and 0 if absent (or nonreactive), for a possible total of 10. A score ≥8 indicates a reassuring test; a score ≤6 indicates a compromised fetus (Landon, 2000). A score of 7 requires retesting in 3 days.

Intrapartum Care

Pregestational and Gestational Diabetes

Nursing care of women with diabetes in labor requires knowledge of obstetrics and medical complications of diabetes. The nurse should obtain the woman's comprehensive and detailed obstetric and diabetes history on admission. Special attention should be given to a history of complications of labor and delivery, such as shoulder dystocia, macrosomia, prolonged labor, stillbirth and adverse neonatal outcomes. Current findings from antenatal testing should be obtained. Recent ultrasound findings should be reviewed, noting estimated fetal weight, amniotic fluid index and fetal

Table 23. Fetal Surveillance for Women with Diabetes

Gestational Age (weeks)	GDMA1 (diet-controlled)	GDMA2 (insulin-controlled)	Type 1 or 2 (well-controlled, no vascular disease)	Type 1 or 2 (poorly controlled or with vascular disease)
6 to 8			Sonographic estimation of gestational age	Sonographic estimation of gestational age
16 to 19	Maternal serum AFP	Maternal serum AFP	Maternal serum AFP	Maternal serum AFP
20 to 22	High resolution sonography	High resolution sonography	High resolution sonography	High resolution sonography, fetal e chocardiography
26 to 28			Sonographic estimation of fetal growth	Sonographic estimation of fetal growth
28.1 to 28.6	Twice-daily fetal movement counting (FMC)	FMC	FMC	FMC and weekly NST
32		Weekly NST, increase to twice weekly at 34 to 36 weeks	Weekly NST, increase to twice weekly at 34 to 36 weeks	Twice weekly NST or weekly BPP and sonographic estimation of fetal growth
36 to 38	Sonographic estimation of fetal weight, weekly NST	Sonographic estimation of fetal weight	Sonographic estimation of fetal weight	Sonographic estimation of fetal weight
36 to 39				With worsening disease, consider amniocentesis and delivery
39 to 40	Elective delivery if cervix favorable and large-for-gestational-age infant	Elective delivery if cervix favorable and large-for-gestational-age infant	Elective delivery without amniocentesis	Elective delivery without amniocentesis

Adapted from Kendrick, 2001

position. Table 24 identifies information about the woman's diabetes history to be reviewed by the nurse.

Blood glucose levels during labor should be maintained between 80 mg/dL and 120 mg/dL (plasma), or 70 mg/dL and 110 mg/dL (whole blood or capillary) (Homko, 1998). Avoidance of maternal hyperglycemia is critical to minimize the development of neonatal hypoglycemia. For women with pregestational diabetes or gestational diabetes controlled by insulin, the nurse should assess blood glucose at the bedside every 1 to 2 hours, with an initial laboratory assessment obtained on admission. Laboratory correlation of blood glucose to capillary bedside testing should be done every 8 hours. Women with GDM controlled by diet do not require as frequent assessment of blood glucose in labor and should be tested every 2 to 4 hours. The nurse

Table 24. Diabetes History

- Diabetes type and classification
- Microvascular complications, including retinopathy, nephropathy and autonomic neuropathy
  - Results of most recent ophthalmology examination
  - Hypertension and medications
  - Results of most recent 24-hour urine for protein and creatinine and serum electrolytes
  - History of orthostatic hypotension
- Antenatal diabetes complications of DKA and hypoglycemia
- Glucose level that precipitates symptoms of hypoglycemia
- Glucose log and self-management diary
- Results of most recent A1C
- Meter type and technique for sampling
- Insulin regimen with time, amount, type of last insulin dose, preferred injection site and regional rotation
- Last food intake

All women with type 1 diabetes require glucose and insulin during labor.

should check urinary ketones with each void, or every 4 hours if blood glucose is within target range. Ketones should be checked when blood glucose values exceed 200 mg/dL. Moderate or large amounts of ketones should alert the nurse to the possibility of starvation or impending ketoacidosis; the nurse should notify the physician to determine if serum ketones should be obtained. Because the presence of ketones may indicate infection, the nurse should observe the woman for signs and symptoms of infection and monitor her temperature. Fever may indicate dehydration or infection.

The intravenous fluid of choice for women with diabetes during labor is based on blood glucose. Intravenous access should be established early to assure adequate hydration and a route for intravenous administration of insulin. All women with type 1 diabetes require glucose and insulin during labor. Women with GDM and type 2 diabetes may not require insulin, but they should be monitored closely. If the blood glucose on admission is ≤70 mg/dL (capillary), an intravenous solution containing 5 percent dextrose should be initiated at a rate of 100 ml/hour to 125 ml/hour. A blood glucose between 70 mg/dL and 110 mg/dL requires administration of a non-glucose-containing solution, such as 0.9 percent sodium chloride or normal saline. Insulin is required when the blood glucose reaches 110 mg/dL by capillary determination and 120 mg/dL by venous plasma determination. Insulin may be given subcutaneously or intravenously per institution protocol or physician preference. The insulin should be titrated to glycemic response to maintain blood glucose levels in the target range. Initial dosages of intravenous insulin are in the range of 1 to 2 units/hour. The nurse should administer the insulin admixture and intravenous glucose via a controlled infusion device after flushing the polyvinyl tubing. When administering insulin via the subcutaneous route, the morning dose of insulin should be decreased by half (Moore, 1999). The nurse should monitor blood glucose levels and administer 2 to 5 units to maintain blood glucose in the target range. Some women may opt to continue to use their

Hypoglycemia in labor can be avoided with continuous nursing assessment.

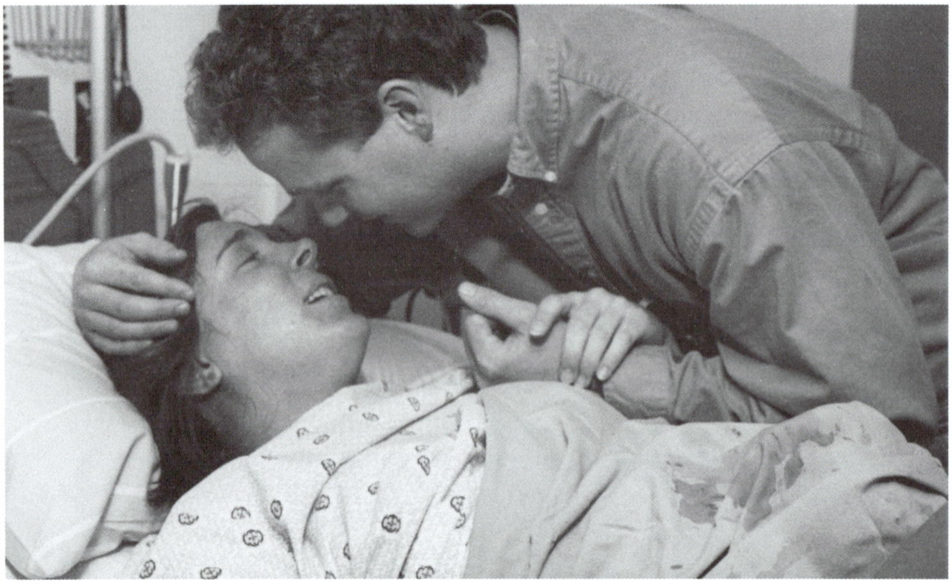

insulin pump during labor; nurses caring for these women should be familiar with use of the pump. Glycemia usually can be maintained with a low, hourly basal rate similar to the prelabor basal rate, with boluses for blood glucose levels >150 mg/dL.

Women with vascular disease who are fluid-restricted should have insulin admixed in a concentrated ratio to reduce the amount of fluid infused. Total intravenous intake should be monitored closely with output and should be maintained at 70 ml/hour (Kendrick, 2001). Closer surveillance of blood glucose in women with nephropathy is required due to the unpredictable action of insulin that occurs as a result of renal catabolism. These women require a lower dose of insulin to achieve euglycemia. Non-glucose-containing solutions should be administered at a slower rate when prehydration is required for conduction anesthesia or for fluid boluses to avoid fluid overload or hyperglycemia (Kendrick, 2001).

Nurses should be alert to signs and symptoms of hypoglycemia. Dextrose in concentrated solutions (10 percent and 50 percent) to treat hypoglycemia in labor should be immediately available. In the presence of hypoglycemia (60 mg/dL capillary or 70 mg/dL plasma), intravenous insulin should be discontinued and 300 ml of 5 percent dextrose infused over 10 to 15 minutes, unless the woman is fluid-restricted (Kendrick, 1999). With fluid restriction, 10 ml of 50 percent dextrose can be administered. The nurse should check blood glucose every 5 minutes during treatment, then every 15 minutes until the blood glucose reaches 120 mg/dL (plasma) or 110 mg/dL (capillary), at which time the insulin infusion should be resumed at a reduced dosage. If the woman loses consciousness, the nurse immediately should notify the physician and rapidly infuse a 50 percent solution of dextrose over 5 to 10 minutes (Kendrick, 1999). If an insulin pump is utilized during labor, the nurse should be familiar with its operation and suspend delivery of insulin with hypoglycemia. Disconnecting the lower connection on the CSII tubing allows for quick release. Hypoglycemia in labor can be avoided with continuous nursing assessment.

Women with diabetes usually do not go into spontaneous labor but are scheduled to deliver by induction or scheduled cesarean. Indications for a scheduled cesarean without labor include untreated proliferative retinopathy, macrosomia >4,500 g or fetal distress. Women with diabetes who have had a cesarean delivery have a lower success rate at vaginal birth (Blackwell et al., 2000; Coleman, Randall, Graves & Lindsay, 2001). Further study in this area is needed to determine safety issues for women with diabetes who desire a vaginal birth after a previous cesarean. Table 25 identifies options for insulin management for labor induction or scheduled cesarean. Nurses should follow hospital procedures for management of cervical ripening, induction or cesarean.

The nurse should evaluate fetal status continuously for evidence of fetal stress or distress. The nurse should be alert to labor progress abnormalities that may indicate cephalopelvic disproportion. The incidence of macrosomia and shoulder dystocia are much higher in women with diabetes, and nurses should be prepared for assisted delivery. Although sonographic measures of estimated fetal weights to diagnose macrosomia are not accurate in predicting which infants will have shoulder dystocia or brachial plexus injury with vaginal birth, cesarean birth rates have increased (Combs, Rosenn, Miodovnik & Siddiqi, 2000; Landon, 2000). Measures of fetal abdominal circumference have been studied to better predict the macrosomic infant (Al-Inany, Alaa, Momtaz & Abdel Badii, 2001; Gilby, Williams & Spellacy, 2000). Fetal truncal asymmetry, when compared to the biparietal diameter of the fetal head, directly correlates to macrosomia and shoulder dystocia (Cohen, Penning, Ansley, Porto & Garite, 1999). Because macrosomia may be predicted in the infant of the mother with diabetes, intrapartum nurses must always consider the possibility and be prepared. This consideration is even more pertinent in obese women with gestational diabetes (Dang, Homko & Reece, 2000).

There are no pain relief methods that are contraindicated in women with diabetes unless there are other medical complications, such as hypertension with coagulation abnormalities.

The incidence of macrosomia and shoulder dystocia are much higher in women with diabetes, and nurses should be prepared for assisted delivery.

Table 25. Insulin Management Options for Labor Induction or Scheduled Cesarean

Condition	Action
GDM	Omit morning dose and schedule for early morning admission.
Type 2 DM	Omit morning dose and schedule for early morning admission.
Type 1	Take intermediate-acting insulin only and schedule for early morning admission. OR Reduce morning dosage of intermediate and rapid-acting insulin by half. OR Omit morning dose and schedule admission 1 hour before usual rising time, beginning glucose and insulin based on blood glucose.

The continual presence of the nurse during labor provides support and reassurance that the woman's diabetes and labor are being monitored closely.

The woman should receive education about pain relief options, and she should choose her pain relief method. Poorly controlled pain in labor releases counterregulatory hormones that antagonize insulin, requiring higher dosages to control blood glucose. Conduction anesthesia during labor, birth or cesarean birth allows for early maternal-infant interaction and for the woman to be alert to signs and symptoms of hypoglycemia.

Psychosocial Issues

The psychosocial changes associated with pregnancy are dramatic. When combined with the stress and demands of a medical complication, such as diabetes, pregnancy can be a major stressor for the woman and her family. Exploring the woman's concerns about labor, birth and her infant is an important aspect of intrapartum nursing care. Ideally, a comprehensive psychosocial evaluation has been performed that identifies the woman's support systems, and the nurse can capitalize on these findings when planning care. However, this is not usually the case, so the nurse must explore the woman's support and coping mechanisms during the intrapartum period.

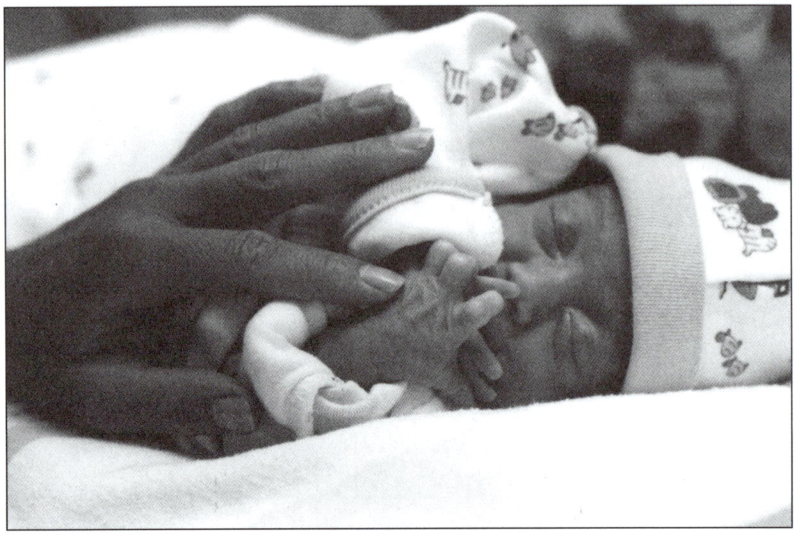

All women need complete explanations of what will occur during childbirth. The woman with diabetes needs to know how her diabetes will be managed during labor—the frequency of blood glucose checks, administration of insulin, her target range for blood glucose in labor and administration of glucose in the fasting state of labor. Some women are fearful and distrustful of staff managing their diabetes. Some may fear that they will become hypoglycemic during labor. The nurse can help relieve these anxieties by discussing diabetes management with the woman so that she feels comfortable relinquishing control to hospital staff.

Women with diabetes often have concerns about the health and well-being of their infants. Women who were unable to achieve a high level of metabolic control during pregnancy may feel guilty and anxious. Perinatal nurses should focus on the positive aspects of the woman's self-care. The nurse should offer reassurance of fetal status whenever possible. If delivery of a preterm infant is anticipated, the nurse should describe neonatal intensive care facilities and provide a tour for the woman and her family, if possible. At the woman's discretion, the nurse should include significant others in discussions about expectations and care.

The diagnosis of fetal macrosomia may cause a woman to fear for her safety and her ability to deliver a large infant vaginally. The nurse should discuss with the woman the possibility of cesarean intervention. The nurse should continuously assess and explain labor progress and fetal response. During labor, the nurse should describe evidence of labor progression and discuss the results of vaginal examinations. The continual presence of the nurse during labor provides support and reassurance that the woman's diabetes and labor are being monitored closely.

Neonatal Considerations

Most infants of mothers with diabetes have an uncomplicated perinatal course, but the risk for adverse outcome is much higher than for infants born to mothers who do not have diabetes. Perinatal nurses caring for women with diabetes during the intrapartum and postpartum periods must be aware of these potential neonatal complications and be prepared to render high-risk care. Full neonatal resuscitation may be required, and all necessary equipment should be checked and immediately available. A neonatal resuscitation team should be present for the birth, when indicated by maternal or fetal status, if not for all births to women with diabetes.

Respiratory Distress Syndrome

The incidence of respiratory distress and respiratory distress syndrome (RDS) has decreased dramatically in the last decade, because infants of women with diabetes are more likely to be delivered after 38 weeks gestation. Increased knowledge about diabetes management has improved perinatal care, decreasing the risk of third-trimester intrauterine fetal death and allowing near-term births. In addition, sophisticated antenatal testing to provide reassurance that the fetus is tolerating the intrauterine environment obviates the need for intervention before fetal lung maturity. However, respiratory distress does occur at a higher incidence in offspring of mothers with diabetes than without. Although the exact underlying mechanism of delayed fetal lung maturation is unknown, the condition is thought to be due to fetal hyperinsulinemia that leads to decreased surfactant production (Schwartz & Teramo, 2000).

An amniocentesis to assess fetal lung maturity is often performed when delivery is indicated before 38 weeks gestation. The lecithin/sphingomyelin (L/S) ratio is not as specific an indicator for fetal lung maturity as the presence of phosphatidylglycerol (PG) (Conway & Langer, 1998; Landon, 2000; Schwartz & Teramo, 2000). Nurses should evaluate the results of the amniocentesis to predict the need for respiratory support after birth. For gestations <38 weeks that have not had an amniocentesis, respiratory difficulty at birth should be anticipated.

Respiratory status should be assessed immediately after birth; the nurse should look for tachypnea, intercostal and subcostal retractions, nasal flaring and expiratory grunting (Jovanovic, 2000). The presence of any of these symptoms indicates respiratory compromise and the need for oxygen therapy. These symptoms may be present at birth or may develop hours later.

Hypoglycemia

Neonatal hypoglycemia is a risk for infants of mothers with diabetes. Maintenance of euglycemia throughout pregnancy and during labor decreases the risk. Neonatal hypoglycemia is caused by fetal hyperinsulinemia in response to maternal hyperglycemia. As soon as the cord is cut, a rapid fall in blood glucose may occur in infants with excessive insulin production. Early feeding may minimize this risk (Jovanovic, 2000; Schwartz & Teramo, 2000). In symptomatic infants who will not feed, intravenous glucose is indicated. To immediately prevent hypoglycemia after birth, the nurse should take steps to prevent hypothermia. Immediately drying the infant and providing care under a radiant warmer will minimize heat loss. Neonatal hypoglycemia generally presents in the first few hours after birth, but it may occur over the next 48 to 72 hours (Schwartz & Teramo, 2000).

The incidence of respiratory distress and respiratory distress syndrome (RDS) has decreased dramatically in the last decade, because infants of women with diabetes are more likely to be delivered after 38 weeks gestation.

Approximately 50 percent of infants born to women with pregestational diabetes develop hypocalcemia during the first 3 days of life

Neonatal blood glucose should be taken within 30 minutes of birth by a glucose meter that is unaffected by hematocrit. If the result is normal, a blood glucose should be obtained every hour until stable. If the level is 40 mg/dL, a venous plasma sample should be obtained. The nurse should continuously observe the infant for signs and symptoms of hypoglycemia, such as abnormal cry, apnea, jitteriness, lethargy, tremors, tachypnea, hypothermia, hypotonia, cyanosis, convulsions and cardiac arrest (Jovanovic, 2000). Most infants with mild to moderate hypoglycemia will be asymptomatic, requiring frequent testing to detect low levels. Long-term sequelae of neonatal hypoglycemia have not been determined.

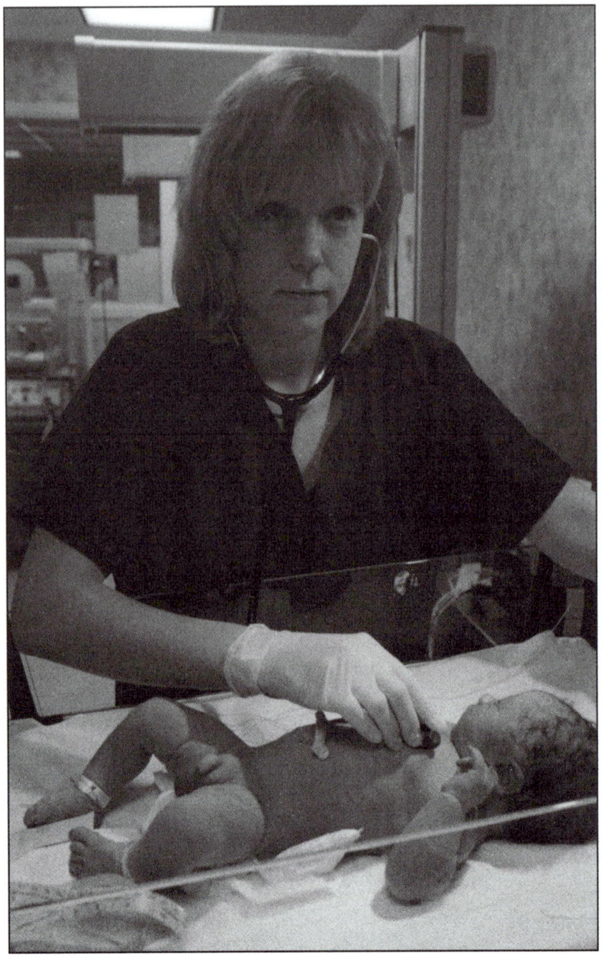

Hypocalcemia and Hypomagnesemia

Approximately 50 percent of infants born to women with pregestational diabetes develop hypocalcemia during the first 3 days of life (Schwartz & Teramo, 2000). Hypocalcemia is defined as 7 mg/dL or <1.75 mmol/L (2 mm) (Schwartz & Teramo, 2000). The severity of hypocalcemia is directly related to the severity of the maternal diabetes. Asphyxia and prematurity also contribute to the development of neonatal hypocalcemia. Pregnancy is considered a hyperparathyroid state that allows transfer of calcium to the fetus, resulting in levels in the fetus that are higher than in the mother. Normally, on the second or third day of life, the neonate produces parathyroid hormone (PTH), in response to falling levels of calcium, to maintain normal calcium levels (Jovanovic, 2000). For unknown reasons, PTH production in infants of mothers with diabetes is suppressed and delayed until the third or fourth day of life (Jovanovic, 2000).

Hypomagnesemia (<1.5 mg/dL) affects 33 percent of infants born to women with pregestational diabetes and, like hypocalcemia, is related to the severity of the maternal diabetes (Schwartz & Teramo, 2000). Clinical symptoms of hypocalcemia and hypomagnesemia are similar to the symptoms of hypoglycemia; serum electrolyte levels are required to provide the diagnosis. Hypomagnesemia reflects the magnesium concentration of the mother (Schwartz & Teramo, 2000). Low magnesium levels may contribute to the development of hypocalcemia by suppressing parathyroid activity. Symptomatic hypocalcemia and hypomagnesemia require intravenous or intramuscular replacement with monitoring of the neonatal heart rate (Jovanovic, 2000).

Hyperbilirubinemia and Polycythemia

Hyperbilirubinemia occurs more frequently in infants of mothers with diabetes than in infants of mothers without diabetes (Jovanovic, 2000). Red blood cell morphology in infants of diabetic mothers does not differ from that of infants born to non-diabetic mothers. Delayed clearance of bilirubin, when measured by pulmonary excretion of carbon monoxide, may be a cause (Stevenson, 1987). Polycythemia, as evidenced by hematocrits >65 percent, affects 20 percent to 40 percent of infants of mothers with diabetes (Jovanovic, 2000). Polycythemia is probably the most important variable in the development of hyperbilrubinemia. Treatment involves the use of partial exchange transfusion through the umbilical vein with plasmanate or 5 percent albumin (Schwartz & Teramo, 2000). Increased oxygen requirements in utero to support anabolic metabolism that results in acidosis may be the underlying mechanism of polycythema (Berkus, Conway & Langer, 1999). Strict glycemic control in the mother nearly eliminates the occurrence of polycythemia (Berkus, Conway & Langer, 1999).

Congenital Defects and Birth Injury

Thirty percent to 40 percent of perinatal deaths in pregnancies complicated by diabetes can be attributed to malformations (Schwartz & Teramo, 2000). There are no specific congenital defects associated with diabetes. Because many congenital defects are detected before birth, nurses can anticipate the immediate needs of the neonate. However, some defects go undetected. Table 26 identifies elements of a comprehensive neonatal assessment. The March of Dimes nursing modules *The Premature Infant: Nursing Assessment and Management* (Vargo & Trotter, 1998) and *Assessment of Risk in the Term Newborn* (Bakewell-Sachs, Shaw & Tashman, 1997) offer comprehensive reviews of neonatal assessment.

Long-Term Prognosis

The immediate neonatal period is not the only time to be concerned about problems in the infant born to the mother with diabetes (Schwartz & Teramo, 2000). Long-term effects of maternal diabetes on growth and development, intellectual functioning and subsequent development of diabetes are areas that require investigation.

Thirty percent to 40 percent of perinatal deaths in pregnancies complicated by diabetes can be attributed to malformations (Schwartz & Teramo, 2000). There are no specific congenital defects associated with diabetes.

Table 26. Elements of a Comprehensive Neonatal Assessment

- Observe the infant for evidence of birth defects
- Observe the infant for evidence of birth injury, including assessment of:
  - Position
  - Body symmetry
  - Range of motion
  - Alertness
- Inspect the head for evidence of cephalohematoma or caput succedaneum
- Measure and document the occipital and frontal circumferences
- Examine the infant for clavicular fracture or brachial plexus injury, especially the infant whose delivery was assisted, has known shoulder dystocia or who weighs >4,000 grams. Assess for decreased or absent arm movement, bruising, crepitus, tenderness or irregularity along the clavicle, which may indicate a fracture.

The postpartum period is an ideal time to stress the importance of continued glycemic control to decrease the risk of long-term complications of diabetes.

In a study of offspring of diabetic mothers (ODM) with pregestational and gestational diabetes, macrosomia observed at birth resolved by 1 year of age but recurred as obesity in childhood and adolescence (Silverman, Rizzo, Cho & Metzger, 1998). Investigators found that the mean BMI in ODM was 24.6 + 5.8 kg/m^2 as compared to 20.9 + 3.4 kg/m^2 in control subjects. Neuropsychological disturbances did not increase in ODM when diabetes in the mother was controlled (Silverman, Rizzo, Cho & Metzger, 1998). Intellectual performance and psychomotor development were impaired in the offspring of mothers who were metabolically unstable. In addition, impaired glucose tolerance was found in 36 percent of ODM and associated with hyperinsulinemia in utero, as detected by amniotic fluid insulin levels (Silverman, Rizzo, Cho & Metzger, 1998). In another study, the incidence of type 2 diabetes in offspring of mothers with pregestational type 2 diabetes was 70 percent in 25- to 34-year-olds (Dabelea, Knowler & Pettitt, 2000). The researchers also found higher rates of obesity.

The development of type 1 diabetes in offspring of mothers with pregestational type 1 diabetes is much lower than that of children of women with type 2 diabetes because the occurrence results from a combination of genetic susceptibility, chronic autoimmune destruction of beta pancreatic cells and an external environmental trigger (Schwartz & Teramo, 2000). The rate of type 1 diabetes in offspring has been reported to be 2 percent to 6 percent, with the highest incidence occurring when the father has type 1 diabetes, rather than the mother (Schwartz & Teramo, 2000). Genetic testing after birth can detect the risk of type 1 diabetes and may allow preventive interventions. The development of gestational diabetes in female offspring of mothers with a history of GDM or type 2 diabetes is 35 percent higher than that of the non-diabetic population (Reece & Homko, 1994).

Postpartum Care

Pregestational and Gestational Diabetes

Most women with pregestational diabetes experience a period of improved insulin sensitivity in the immediate postpartum period due to the dramatic decrease in contrainsulin hormones (Kjos, 2000). Insulin requirements are greatly reduced. In postoperative women, the rate of insulin infusion should be decreased by half after birth until oral intake is tolerated (Kendrick, 2001). Women with type 2 diabetes usually can discontinue insulin after giving birth. Blood glucose levels should be monitored closely in the first 24 hours and insulin given as necessary, and testing should revert to the pre-pregnancy testing pattern. Insulin requirements should be recalculated during the postpartum period for all women with type 1 diabetes and for lactating women with type 2 diabetes. The pre-pregnancy dose may be resumed or a dosage calculated based on postpartum weight. If using postpartum weight, 0.6 U/kg/day should be adequate for achievement of euglycemia (Jovanovic, 2000). Non-lactating women with type 2 diabetes may resume oral anti-diabetes agents.

The postpartum period is an ideal time to stress the importance of continued glycemic control to decrease the risk of long-term complications of diabetes. Most pregnant women with pregestational diabetes strive for metabolic control to improve the health of their unborn infant. Women who are able to achieve metabolic control during pregnancy often realize that they can control their diabetes and attain a better quality of life following pregnancy.

Many are motivated to continue to manage their diabetes comprehensively. If the woman does not have a diabetes specialist as a provider, referral is appropriate to support her efforts to control her disease. The diabetes provider or perinatal diabetes management team should follow up to assess the woman's diabetes management within 3 weeks of hospital discharge.

Glycemia in women with gestational diabetes generally improves soon after birth. Glucose testing is no longer required in women who are not on insulin therapy. However, some women have unrecognized diabetes predating the pregnancy (Kjos, 2000). The ADA (2003d) recommends reclassification testing for diabetes. Testing can be delayed until the 6-week postpartum checkup for non-lactating women and until weaning for lactating women. Table 27 lists diagnostic criteria for diabetes. Since the ADA adopted these stricter criteria in 1997, postpartum diagnosis of diabetes has doubled (Conway & Langer, 1999). Women with impaired fasting glucose (IFG) (between 110 mg/dL and 126 mg/dL) or impaired glucose tolerance (IGT) (2-hour plasma glucose between 140 mg/dL and 200 mg/dL) should be tested annually. An individualized exercise program and medical nutrition therapy should be emphasized to decrease or delay the onset of overt diabetes mellitus in this group of women (ADA, 2003d). The testing interval for women with normal postpartum tests is every 3 years and before conception to allow for preconception detection and intensive management of diabetes (ADA, 2003d).

This risk for developing type 2 diabetes increases with time (Kendrick, 2001). For women with GDM who are more likely to develop type 2 diabetes within 5 years of delivery, risk factors for type 2 diabetes are diagnosis of GDM in the first trimester, obesity and hyperglycemia at the postpartum visit (ADA, 2003d). Postpartum education should include strategies to reduce the risk of developing overt diabetes, such as modest weight reduction and exercise (Kendrick, 2001). The nurse should review with the woman signs and symptoms of hyperglycemia and when to seek testing. Women should also receive counseling about the 70 percent risk for GDM in subsequent pregnancies (Major, de Veciana, Weeks & Morgan, 1998).

Women with pregestational and gestational diabetes require nutrition evaluation before discharge from the hospital to recalculate caloric needs. The non-breastfeeding postpartum woman requires approximately 25 kcal/kg/day, and the breastfeeding woman requires 27 kcal/kg/day (Jovanovic, 2000). Goals of nutrition therapy in the postpartum period are to attain or maintain ideal body weight and meet demands of lactation. The nurse should review weight reduction strategies with non-lactating obese women. Caloric needs to support lactation increase by approximately 500 kcal. Breastfeeding is encouraged for women with diabetes to decrease the risk of diabetes development in offspring (Perez-Bravo et al., 1996; Pettitt, Forman, Hanson, Knowler & Bennett, 1997). In addition, breastfeeding in women with a history of GDM decreases the risk of the development of overt diabetes later in life for the mother (Kjos, Henry, Lee, Buchanan & Mishell, 1993). Hypoglycemia occurs more frequently in lactating women with pregestational diabetes. Adequate calories and fluid intake are necessary to minimize the risk of hypoglycemia; eating a snack immediately before or during breastfeeding reduces this risk. Late night nursing carries the highest risk of hypoglycemia; eating a bedtime snack may minimize this risk.

Breastfeeding is encouraged for women with diabetes to decrease the risk of diabetes development in offspring.

Table 27. Diagnostic Criteria for Diabetes*

Normoglycemia	IFG and IGT	Diabetes Mellitus
FPG <110 mg/dL	FPG between 110 mg/dL and 126 mg/dL (IFG)	FPG >126 mg/dL on two occasions
2-hour plasma glucose <140 mg/dL	2-hour plasma glucose between 140 mg/dL and 200 mg/dL	2-hour plasma glucose >200 mg/dL
		Symptoms of diabetes mellitus and casual plasma glucose >200 mg/dL

FPG=fasting plasma glucose
IFG=impaired fasting glucose
IGT=impaired glucose tolerance
*A diagnosis must be confirmed on a subsequent day for any of the three methods.

Adapted from ADA, 2003d

Contraception

Contraception is an important issue to address in the immediate postpartum period. Table 7 presents an overview of contraceptive options for women with diabetes. Progestin-only oral contraceptives are contraindicated in lactating women with a history of gestational diabetes due to the threefold increased risk for the development of overt diabetes (Kjos et al., 1998). The risk is even higher with prolonged, uninterrupted use. The nurse should re-emphasize the importance of pregnancy planning, preconception glycemic control and the need for contraception. For women with gestational diabetes, contraception is important to prevent conception until their glycemic status is re-evaluated. The woman who does not desire future fertility should explore permanent contraceptive options. Intrauterine devices may increase the risk of infection but can provide prolonged infertility in women who do not desire permanent sterilization. In women with vascular disease who have surgical and anesthetic risks, a vasectomy for the male partner is a safer alternative than a tubal ligation for the woman.

Psychosocial Issues with the High-Risk Neonate

Intensive diabetes management and improved metabolic control have greatly improved outcomes in infants born to women with diabetes, but the risk for adverse outcomes is still present. Some infants require observation and management in neonatal intensive care. In the event of prematurity or congenital defects, the parents may have been prepared for neonatal intensive care by touring the facilities and having their questions and concerns addressed. However, not all admissions can be predicted. The nurse should take every opportunity to relieve parental anxiety. Maternal-infant contact should occur at the earliest and safest opportunity, taking into consideration the mother's and the infant's condition. Photos or videos of the infant provide contact with the infant when face-to-face contact is not possible. Most neonatal intensive care units have social workers who can help new parents adjust to having a sick infant and provide links to appropriate support groups. Parents should participate in caregiving and should be kept informed of the infant's condition. Breastfeeding should be encouraged and a breast pump made available with lactation consultation.

The nurse can explore with the woman any guilty feelings about the infant's condition. The nurse should make referral to a mental health specialist for further evaluation, if necessary. A history of depression warrants more comprehensive assessment because it increases the woman's risk of postpartum depression and may affect her ability to manage her diabetes.

Summary

Women with diabetes have unique needs during the perinatal period that determine healthy outcomes for themselves and their infants. Ideally, for women with pregestational diabetes, this care should begin before conception. Nurses are challenged to provide comprehensive management strategies and education for the woman with diabetes and her family to empower them with the knowledge for self-care during the perinatal period.

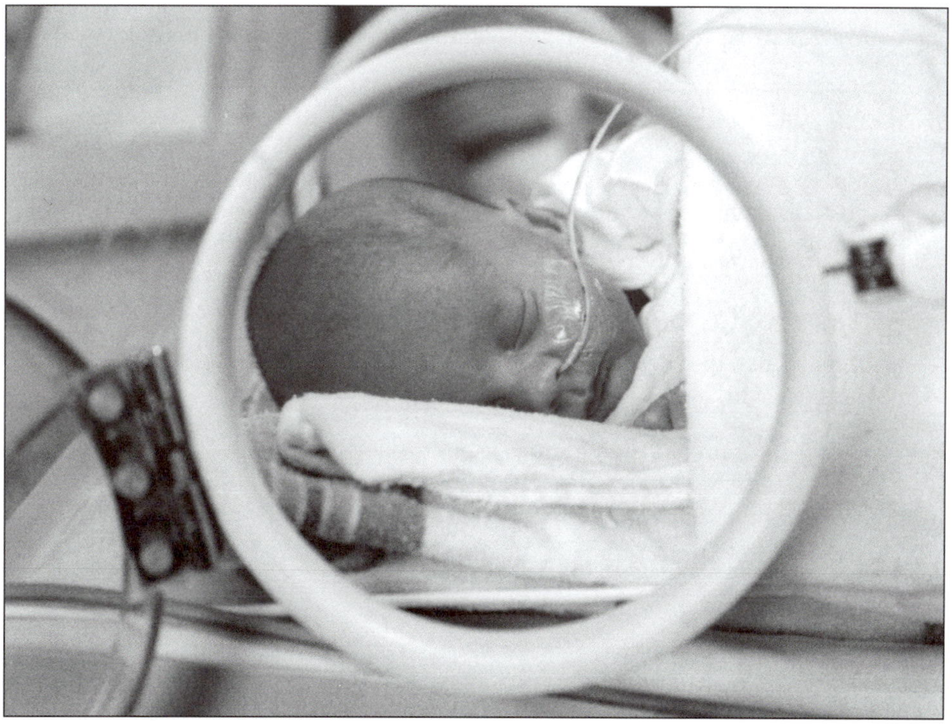

CLINICAL APPLICATION

The following activities will aid the learner in applying concepts presented in this module.

1. Ms. K is 26 weeks gestation and just received her 1-hour glucola test result, which was 210 mg/dL. Her history includes gestational diabetes requiring insulin and the birth of an infant weighing 9 pounds, 4 ounces.

    a. Does Ms. K need further diagnostic testing?

    b. What factors put Ms. K at risk for the development of GDM?

    c. At what point in Ms. K's prenatal care should testing for GDM be obtained?

    d. What laboratory test can determine if Ms. K's hyperglycemia has been present for a while?

    e. What education topics should the nurse discuss with Ms. K?

    f. What fasting and posprandial values define glycemic control in pregnancy?

    g. Ms. K says she read on the Internet that glyburide could be taken during pregnancy to control GDM. How should the nurse address her concern?

    h. What are Ms. K's risks for the development of overt diabetes? Is there anything she can do to decrease this risk?

    i. Ms. K comes in for a prenatal and diabetes management visit at 29 weeks gestation and does not bring her blood glucose meter with her. She states she hasn't been taking her blood glucose consistently. What should the nurse's approach be? Are there any tests that might be indicated for the fetus?

    j. If Ms. K had undiagnosed pre-existing diabetes, what potential risks exist for her child?

    k. Was Ms. K's previous child macrosomic?

    l. What are the risks for the infant at birth with macrosomia?

    m. When Ms. K delivers, the nurse should observe the newborn for what neonatal risks?

    n. What are the long-term risks for Ms. K's child?

2. Ms. D has had type 1 diabetes for 5 years. She comes to the emergency room at 26 weeks gestation with nausea and vomiting, abdominal pain, rapid respirations, fruity breath and mild confusion.

    a. What diagnosis should the nurse suspect?

    b. What laboratory assessments should be made immediately?

    c. What infection in pregnant women is associated with the development of DKA?

d. What laboratory values are diagnostic of DKA?

e. What is the most important intervention in the treatment of DKA?

f. What is the usual initial insulin dose for pregnant women experiencing DKA?

g. The EFM strip from Ms. D's fetus shows evidence of late decelerations. Should the nurse prepare for a cesarean?

h. The EFM strip also shows evidence of frequent uterine contractions, and Ms. D's cervix is 1 to 2 centimeters dilated. What is the safest tocolytic to use?

i. What sick day guidelines should Ms. D incorporate into her self-care regimen to prevent the development of DKA?

j. What education should the nurse give Ms. D when she is discharged from the hospital?

GROUP DISCUSSION ITEMS

The following discussion items will aid the learner in applying concepts presented in this module.

1. Survey the resources available in your community that provide diabetes education with a perinatal component.

2. Identify grief support groups available for parents who have lost a child either by miscarriage, stillbirth or neonatal death.

3. Determine resources available for women with diabetes who are non-English speaking or hearing or visually impaired.

4. Evaluate diabetes in pregnancy policies, procedures and protocols in your institution to determine accuracy and comprehensiveness.

5. Determine if women with diabetes receive multidisciplinary care in your community.

6. List preconception factors that improve outcomes in women with diabetes.

INDEPENDENT STUDY TEST

Diabetes in Pregnancy, 3rd Edition

To receive continuing education credit for completion of this module via independent study, record answers to the following questions on the Independent Study Application and submit it to March of Dimes for grading. Submission instructions are listed on the application.

1. Type 1 diabetes mellitus is associated with:
   A. Insulin resistance
   B. A pancreatic secretory defect
   C. An inappropriate response to insulin
   D. Autoimmunity directed at pancreatic beta cells

2. Proliferative retinopathy, which can worsen during pregnancy, is associated with:
   A. Autoimmunity
   B. Neovascularization
   C. Macrovascular changes
   D. Autonomic dysfunction

3. When monitoring for diabetic ketoacidosis during pregnancy, the nurse should assess the woman for:
   A. Hypotension
   B. Paresthesias
   C. Hunger
   D. Pallor

4. When administering insulin intravenously to a woman in diabetic ketoacidosis, it is important for the nurse to:
   A. Discontinue the infusion as soon as ketoacidosis resolves.
   B. Assess for the development of hyperkalemia.
   C. Dilute the insulin in Lactated Ringer's Solution.
   D. Lower the blood glucose level slowly.

5. Overall glycemic control in a pregnant woman with diabetes mellitus can best be assessed by:
   A. Measuring blood glucose levels several times a day
   B. Performing a biophysical profile (BPP) each trimester
   C. Determining compliance via weekly telephone contacts
   D. Monitoring the glycosylated hemoglobin every 4 weeks

6. Appropriate sick day management during periods of illness when solid food is not tolerated includes:
   A. Reducing the usual insulin dose
   B. Notifying the practitioner of blood glucose levels >130 mg/dL
   C. Drinking liquids equal to the carbohydrate value of the prescribed diet
   D. Monitoring the blood glucose level every 6 hours when vomiting occurs

7. When monitoring a woman with diabetes mellitus, which adaptation may indicate mild hypoglycemia?
   A. Confusion
   B. Tachycardia
   C. Blurred vision
   D. Extreme fatigue

8. The nurse understands that a woman will be diagnosed with gestational diabetes when two laboratory tests reveal:
   A. Glucose challenge test result >120 mg/dL
   B. Fasting plasma glucose result >126 mg/dL
   C. Random plasma glucose result >160 mg/dL
   D. Three-hour oral glucose tolerance result >130 mg/dL

9. Women with a history of gestational diabetes mellitus should have appropriate medical supervision because they are at risk for developing:
   A. Infertility
   B. Hypocalcemia
   C. Type 2 diabetes mellitus
   D. Severe postpartum depression

10. To best monitor for intrauterine growth retardation (IUGR) in the fetus of a woman with diabetes mellitus, the nurse should plan for:
    A. A contraction stress test in the second trimester
    B. An amniocentesis by the 36th week gestation
    C. Serial ultrasounds beginning in the third trimester
    D. Maternal serum alpha-fetoprotein testing before 16 weeks gestation

11. A pregnant woman with diabetes mellitus who has peripheral vascular disease should be taught to:
    A. Inspect the feet daily.
    B. Cut the toenails in a rounded shape monthly.
    C. Apply moisturizer between the toes weekly.
    D. Warm the feet with a heating pad whenever they get cold.

12. When teaching a woman with diabetes mellitus about barrier methods of contraceptives, the nurse should tell the woman that they may increase the risk for:
    A. Cardiovascular disease
    B. Urinary tract infections
    C. Thrombophlebitis
    D. Pelvic infection

13. Self-monitoring of blood glucose is essential at bedtime to help minimize:
    A. Nocturnal hypoglycemia
    B. Starvation ketosis
    C. Urine ketone testing
    D. Hypoglycemia unawareness

14. The nurse knows that a pregnant woman with type 1 diabetes mellitus understands teaching about medication when the woman says:
    A. "I should be taking just human insulins."
    B. "I may eventually need to take Humalog lispro insulin."
    C. "I can use intermediate-acting insulin in my insulin pump."
    D. "I will need to switch to an oral antidiabetic medication while pregnant."

INDEPENDENT STUDY APPLICATION

Diabetes in Pregnancy, 3rd Edition

To receive continuing education credit for registered nurses and certified nurse-midwives via independent study of *Diabetes in Pregnancy*, 3rd Edition:

1. Complete the registration information.
2. Legibly write the letter of the answer for each question in the spaces provided.
3. Sign and date the application.
4. Return the application and the tear-out self-mailer evaluation to: Nursing Modules, March of Dimes, 1275 Mamaroneck Avenue, White Plains, NY 10605.

The March of Dimes will notify you of your results within 8 weeks of receiving your completed test. If you receive a passing score (70 percent), you will receive a certificate of completion indicating the amount of continuing education earned. If your score is less than 70 percent, you will be given a second opportunity to pass the test.

This continuing education activity was approved by the New York State Nurses Association, an accredited approver by the American Nurses Credentialing Center's Commission on Accreditation. **It has been approved for 6.8 contact hours for registered nurses.** The March of Dimes is also approved as a continuing education provider by the State of California Board of Registered Nursing, Provider #CEP-111444.

This module is also approved for .45 continuing education units (CEUs) for certified nurse-midwives (CNMs) by the American College of Nurse-Midwives (ACNM) (program #2003/087). ACNM approval expires 10/15/05. CNMs should verify the module's approval status at marchofdimes.com/nursing if used after the expiration date.

REGISTRATION INFORMATION

Name ____________________

Credentials ____________________

Address ____________________

City ____________________ State __________ ZIP __________

Telephone ____________________ Fax ____________________

E-mail ____________________

INDEPENDENT STUDY TEST ANSWERS

1. ______	5. ______	9. ______	13. ______
2. ______	6. ______	10. ______	14. ______
3. ______	7. ______	11. ______	
4. ______	8. ______	12. ______	

Signature ____________________ Date __________

CHECKLIST FOR MAILING

☐ Completed (and signed) application

☐ Completed evaluation

MARCH OF DIMES NURSING MODULE EVALUATION

Diabetes in Pregnancy, 3rd Edition

Please remove and complete the evaluation, fold and staple it to reveal the postage-paid portion, and post it in a U.S. mailbox. (Note: Independent study takers can submit the evaluation with their tests for grading; group study participants can give the evaluation to their facilitator.) Thank you in advance for your time. Your responses are important to us as we plan additional continuing education activities.

1. State(s) in which you currently practice

____

2. Professional identification *(Check all that apply.)*

- ☐ Registered nurse
- ☐ Nurse practitioner
- ☐ Clinical nurse specialist
- ☐ Certified nurse-midwife
- ☐ Childbirth educator
- ☐ Nursing student
- ☐ Other *(Please identify.)* ____________________

3. Educational degree(s) *(Check all that apply.)*

- ☐ Diploma nurse
- ☐ Associate degree
- ☐ Baccalaureate in nursing
- ☐ Baccalaureate in other field *(Please identify.)*

____

- ☐ Master's in nursing
- ☐ Master's in other field *(Please identify.)*

____

- ☐ Doctorate in nursing
- ☐ Doctorate in other field *(Please identify.)*

____

4. Area(s) of certification

____

5. Current employment setting

- ☐ Hospital
- ☐ Clinic
- ☐ Private practice
- ☐ Other *(Please identify.)* ____________________

6. Type of work

- ☐ Administration
- ☐ Education—academic/clinical
- ☐ Clinical practice
- ☐ Public health
- ☐ Other *(Please identify.)* ____________________

7. Length of time employed in the health care field

- ☐ <1 year
- ☐ 1 to 2 years
- ☐ 2 to 10 years
- ☐ 10 to 20 years
- ☐ >20 years

8. How did you find out about this module?

- ☐ March of Dimes chapter
- ☐ March of Dimes National Office
- ☐ March of Dimes Web site
- ☐ Conference
- ☐ Place of employment
- ☐ Peer/Colleague recommendation
- ☐ Other *(Please identify.)* ____________________

____

9. Have you used other nursing modules?

☐ Yes ☐ No ☐ Unsure

10. If you are a prior module user, how many modules have you used? ______

11. If you are a prior module user, when was the last time you used a module?

- ☐ <1 month ago
- ☐ 1 month to 1 year ago
- ☐ 1 to 2 years ago
- ☐ >2 years ago

12. How did you use this module?

- ☐ Independent study for continuing education credit
- ☐ Group study for continuing education credit
- ☐ As a learning tool without continuing education credit
- ☐ Other *(Please identify.)* ____________________

____

13. Time required to read the module and complete the independent study test, if applicable

____hours ____minutes ☐ Not applicable

14. Time required to read the module and participate in the facilitated group study, if applicable

____hours ____minutes ☐ Not applicable

Rate each of the following:

	Excellent	Very Good	Good	Fair	Poor	N/A
15. Cognitive objectives						
16. Relationship of cognitive objectives to the overall purpose of the module						
17. Expected practice outcomes						
18. Key concepts						
19. Content						
20. Clinical application						
21. Group discussion items						
22. References						
23. Supplementary materials						
24. Overall quality of the module						
25. Effectiveness of the module as teaching/learning material						
26. Effectiveness of module as a means to increase awareness of the issue/topic						

(Continued on other side)

MARCH OF DIMES NURSING MODULE EVALUATION

27. Which may change as a result of completing this module?
- ☐ Your attitude
- ☐ Your knowledge base
- ☐ Your skill level
- ☐ Other *(Please identify.)* ______________________

28. How might your use of the nursing process be affected by the module?
- ☐ Improved data collection
- ☐ Improved client assessment
- ☐ Improved accuracy in nursing diagnoses
- ☐ Improved discharge planning
- ☐ Improved (more appropriate) nursing interventions
- ☐ Improved evaluation of nursing care
- ☐ Other *(Please identify.)* ______________________

29. Would you recommend this module to a colleague?
☐ Yes ☐ No ☐ Unsure

30. How can the module be improved?

____

31. Suggestions for future module topics

____

32. Other comments

____

Fold Line

NO POSTAGE NECESSARY IF MAILED IN THE UNITED STATES

BUSINESS REPLY MAIL

FIRST CLASS • PERMIT NO. 2000 • WHITE PLAINS, NY

POSTAGE WILL BE PAID BY ADDRESSEE

March of Dimes Birth Defects Foundation
Education Services
1275 Mamaroneck Avenue
White Plains, NY 10602-9989

Fold Line

FOR FACILITATORS ONLY

1. Number of participants attending the study

____

2. Location of the study

____

3. Date of the study

____

4. Length time for the study

____

5. When was the study held?
- ☐ During compensated on-duty time
- ☐ As an overtime (paid) activity
- ☐ On noncompensated time
- ☐ Other *(Please identify.)* ______________________

6. Reasons for the group study *(Check all that apply.)*
- ☐ To offer/obtain continuing education credit
- ☐ To cross-train staff
- ☐ To enhance clinical skills
- ☐ Other *(Please identify.)* ______________________

7. Did you offer/obtain continuing education credit for the module from the March of Dimes?
☐ Yes ☐ No

8. How could the group study process be improved?

____

REFERENCES

Agarwal, M.M., Hughes, P.F., Punnose, J. & Ezimokhai, M. (2000). Fasting plasma glucose as a screening test for gestational diabetes in a multi-ethnic, high-risk population. *Diabetes Medicine, 17*, 720-726.

Ahroni, J.H. (2001). Diabetic foot care and education. In M.J. Franz (Ed.), *Core Curriculum in Diabetes Education: Diabetes and Complications* (4th edition) (pp. 4-86). Chicago: American Association of Diabetes Educators.

Al-Inany, H., Alaa, N., Momtaz, M. & Abdel Badii, M. (2001). Intrapartum prediction of macrosomia: Accuracy of abdominal circumference estimation. *Gynecologic and Obstetric Investigation, 51*, 116-119.

American College of Obstetricians & Gynecologists (ACOG). (1994). Exercise during pregnancy and the postpartum period (ACOG Technical Bulletin #189). *International Journal of Gynaecology and Obstetrics, 45*, 65-70.

American College of Obstetricians & Gynecologists (ACOG). (2001). Gestational diabetes (ACOG Practice Bulletin #30). *Obstetics & Gynecology, 98*, 525-538.

American Diabetes Association (ADA). (2003a). Continuous subcutaneous insulin infusion. *Diabetes Care, 26*(Suppl. 1), S125.

American Diabetes Association (ADA). (2003b). Diabetic nephropathy. *Diabetes Care, 26*(Suppl. 1), S94-S98.

American Diabetes Association (ADA). (2003c). Diabetic retinopathy. *Diabetes Care, 26*(Suppl. 1), S99-S102.

American Diabetes Association (ADA). (2003d). Gestational diabetes mellitus. *Diabetes Care, 26*(Suppl. 1), S103-S105.

American Diabetes Association (ADA). (2003e). Hyperglycemic crisis in patients with diabetes mellitus. *Diabetes Care, 26*(Suppl. 1), S109-S117.

American Diabetes Association (ADA). (2003f). Physical activity/exercise and diabetes mellitus. *Diabetes Care, 26*(Suppl. 1), S73-S77.

American Diabetes Association (ADA). (2003g). Preconception care of women with diabetes. *Diabetes Care, 26*(Suppl. 1), S91-S98.

American Diabetes Association (ADA). (1994). Self monitoring of blood glucose. *Diabetes Care, 17*, 81-6.

American Diabetes Association (ADA). (2003h). Standards of medical care for patients with diabetes mellitus. *Diabetes Care, 26*(Suppl. 1), S33-S50.

Artal, R. & Sherman, C. (1999). Exercise during pregnancy. *The Physician and Sports Medicine, 27*(8), 51-57.

Atilano, L.C., Lee-Parritz, A., Lieberman, E., Cohen, A.P. & Barbieri, R.L. (1999). Alternative methods of diagnosing gestational diabetes mellitus. *American Journal of Obstetrics & Gynecology, 181*, 1158-1161.

REFERENCES

Bakewell-Sachs, S., Shaw, V.D. & Tashman, A.L. (1997). *Assessment of risk in the term newborn.* White Plains, NY: March of Dimes.

Bar, J., Chen, R., Schoenfeld, A., Orvieto, R., Yaha, J., Ben-Rafael, Z. & Hod, M. (1999). Pregnancy outcome in patients with insulin-dependent diabetes mellitus and diabetic nephropathy treated with ACE inhibitors before pregnancy. *Journal of Pediatric Endocinology and Metabolism, 12*, 659-665.

Bartha, J.L., Martinez-Del-Fresno, P. & Comino-Delgado, R. (2000). Gestational diabetes mellitus diagnosed during early pregnancy. *American Journal of Obstetrics and Gynecology, 182*, 346-350.

Berkus, M.D., Conway, D. & Langer, O. (1999). The large fetus. *Clinical Obstetrics and Gynecology, 42*, 766-784.

Betschart, J. (2001). Diabetes during childhood and adolescence. In M.J. Franz (Ed.), *A Core Curriculum of Diabetes Education: Diabetes in the Life Cycle and Research* (4th ed.) (pp. 3-25). Chicago: American Association of Diabetes Educators.

Bevier, W.C., Fischer, R. & Jovanovic, L. (1999). Treatment of women with an abnormal glucose challenge test (but a normal oral glucose tolerance test) decreases the prevalence of macrosomia. *American Journal of Perinatology, 16*, 269-275.

Bhattacharyya, A., Brown, S., Hughes, S. & Vice, P.A. (2001). Insulin lispro and regular insulin in pregnancy. *QGM 94*, 255-260.

Biastre, S.A. (2001). Gestational diabetes mellitus. In M.J. Franz (Ed.), *A Core Curriculum of Diabetes Education: Diabetes in the Life Cycle and Research* (4th ed.) (pp. 73-100). Chicago: American Association of Diabetes Educators.

Biesenbach, G., Grafinger, P., Zazgornik, J. & Helmut, S. (2000). Perinatal complications and 3-year follow-up of infants of diabetic mothers with diabetic nephropathy stage IV. *Renal Failure, 22*, 573-580.

Bjorklund, A., Adamson, U., Andrasson, K., Carlstrom, K., Hennen, G., Igout, A., Lins, P.E. & Westgren, M. (1998). Hormonal counter regulation and subjective symptoms during induced hypoglycemia in insulin dependent diabetes mellitus patients during and after pregnancy. *Acta Obstetricia et Gynecolica Scandinavia, 77*, 625-634.

Blackwell, S.C., Hassan, S.S., Wolfe, H.M., Michaelson, J., Berry, S.M. & Sorokin, Y. (2000). Vaginal birth after cesarean in the diabetic gravida. *Journal of Reproductive Medicine, 45*, 987-990.

Breedlove, G.K. & Schorfheide, A.M. (2001). *Adolescent pregnancy* (2nd Ed.). White Plains, NY: March of Dimes.

Buchanan, T.A. & Coustan, D.R. (1995). Diabetes mellitus. In G.N. Burrows & T.F. Ferris (Eds.), *Medical Complications During Pregnancy* (4th Ed.). Philadelphia: W.B. Saunders.

REFERENCES

Bung, P., Artal, R., Khodiguian, N. & Kjos, S. (1991). Exercise in gestational diabetes. An optional therapeutic approach? *Diabetes, 40*(Suppl. 1), 182-185.

Buschman Gemma, P. & Arnold, J. (2002). *Loss and grieving in pregnancy and the first year of life: A caring resource for nurses.* White Plains, NY: March of Dimes.

Butte, N.F. (2000). Carbohydrate and lipid metabolism in pregnancy: Normal compared to gestational diabetes mellitus. *American Journal of Clinical Nutrition, 71*(Suppl. 5), 1256S-1261S.

Carpenter, M.W. (2000). The role of exercise in pregnant women with diabetes mellitus. *Clinical Obstetrics and Gynecology, 43*, 56-64.

Centers for Disease Control and Prevention (CDC) (1998). Diabetes during pregnancy, United States, 1993-1995. *MMWR, 47*, 408-414.

Chauhan, S.P. & Perry, K.G., Jr. (1995). Management of diabetic ketoacidosis in the obstetric patient. *Obstetrics and Gynecology Clinics of North America, 22*, 143-155.

Cohen, B.F., Penning, S., Ansley, D., Porto, M. & Garite, T. (1999). The incidence and severity of shoulder dystocia correlates with sonographic measurement of asymmetry in patients with diabetes. *American Journal of Perinatology, 16*, 197-201.

Coleman, T.L., Randall, H., Graves, W. & Lindsay, M. (2001). Vaginal birth after cesarean among women with gestational diabetes. *American Journal of Obstetrics and Gynecology, 184*, 1104-1107.

Combs, C.A., Rosenn, B., Kitzmiller, J.L., Khoury, J.C., Wheeler, B.C. & Miodovnik, M. (1993). Early-pregnancy proteinuria in diabetes related to preeclampsia. *Obstetrics and Gynecology, 82*, 802-807.

Combs, C.A., Rosenn, B., Miodovnik, M. & Siddiqi, T.A. (2000). Sonographic EFW and macrosomia: Is ther an optimum formula to predict diabetic fetal macrosomia? *Journal of Maternal Fetal Medicine, 9*, 55-61.

Conway, D.L. & Langer, O. (1998). Optmal timing and mode of delivery in gestational diabetic pregnancy. *Prenatal Neonatal Medicine, 3*, 555-562.

Conway, D.L. & Langer, O. (1999). Effects of new criteria for type 2 diabetes on the rate of postpartum glucose intolerance in women with gestational diabetes. *American Journal of Obstetrics and Gynecology, 81*, 610-614.

Coonrod, B.A. & Ernst, K.L. (2001). Nephropathy. In M.J. Franz (Ed.), *A Core Curriculum of Diabetes Education: Diabetes and Complications* (4th ed.) (pp. 153-88). Chicago: American Association of Diabetes Educators.

Cullen, M.T., Reece, E.A., Homko, C.J. & Sivan, E. (1996). The changing presentations of diabetic ketoacidosis during pregnancy. *American Journal of Perinatology, 13*, 449-451.

Cundy, T., Gamble, G., Townend, K., Henley, P.G., MacPherson, P. & Roberts, A.B. (2000). Perinatal mortality in type 2 diabetes. *Diabetic Medicine, 182*, 33-39.

Dabelea, D., Knowler, W.C. & Pettitt, D. J. (2000). Effect of diabetes in pregnancy on offspring: Follow-up research in Pima Indians. *Journal of Maternal Fetal Medicine, 9*, 83-88.

Dang, K., Homko, C.J. & Reece, E.A. (2000). Factors associated with fetal macrosomia in offspring of gestational diabetic women. *Journal of Maternal Fetal Medicine, 9*, 114-117.

Davidson, M.B. (2001). Hyperglycemia. In M.J. Franz (Ed.), *A Core Curriculum of Diabetes Education: Diabetes and Complications* (4th ed.) (pp. 21-42). Chicago: American Association of Diabetes Educators.

Delamater, A.M., Jacobson, A.M., Anderson, B., Cox, D., Fisher, L., Lustman, P., Rubin, R. & Wysocki, T. (2001). Psychosocial therapies in diabetes: Report of the Diabetes Therapies Working Group. *Diabetes Care, 24*, 1286-1292.

Diabetes Control and Complications Trial (DCCT) Research Group. (1993). The effect of intensive treatment of diabetes on the development and progression of long-term complications in insulin-dependent diabetes mellitus. *New England Journal of Medicine, 329*, 977-986.

Dye, T.D., Knox, K.L., Artal, R., Aubry, R. & Wojtowycz, M.A. (1997). Physical activity, obesity, and diabetes in pregnancy. *American Journal of Epidemiology, 146*, 961-965.

Ekbom, P., Damm, P., Feldt-Rasmussen, B., Feldt-Rasmussen, U., Molvig, J. & Mathiesen, E.R. (2001). Pregnancy outcome in type 1 diabetic women with microalbuminuria. *Diabetes Care, 24*, 1739-1744.

Expert Committee on the Diagnosis and Classification of Diabetes Mellitus. (2003). Report of the expert committee on the diagnosis and classification of diabetes mellitus. *Diabetes Care, 26*(Suppl. 1), S5-S20.

Feldman, E.L., Stevens, M.J., Thomas, P.K., Brown, M.B., Canal, N. & Greene, D.A. (1994). A practical two-step quantitative clinical and electrophysiological assessment for the diagnosis and staging of diabetic neuropathy. *Diabetes Care, 17*, 1281-1289.

Fineberg, S.E., Bergenstal, R.M., Bernstein, R.M., Laffel, L.M. & Schwartz, S.L. (2001). Use of an automated device for alternative site blood glucose monitoring. *Diabetes Care, 24*, 1217-1220.

Franz, M.J. (2001). Medical nutrition therapy. In M.J. Franz (Ed.), *A Core Curriculum of Diabetes Education: Diabetes Management Therapies* (4th ed.) (pp. 3-52). Chicago: American Association of Diabetes Educators.

Funnel, M.M. & Feldman, E.L. (2001). Diabetic neuropathy. In M.J. Franz (Ed.), *A Core Curriculum of Diabetes Education: Diabetes and Complications* (4th ed.) (pp. 191-220). Chicago: American Association of Diabetes Educators.

REFERENCES

Gabbe, S.G. (2001). New concepts and applications in the use of the insulin pump during pregnancy. *Journal of Maternal Fetal Medicine, 9*, 42-45.

Gemma, P.B. & Arnold, J. (2002). *Loss and grieving in pregnancy and the first year of life: A caring resource for nurses.* White Plains, NY: March of Dimes.

Gilby, J.R., Williams, M.C. & Spellacy, W.N. (2000). Fetal abdominal circumference measurements of 35 and 38 cm as predictors of macrosomia: A risk factor for shoulder dystocia. *Journal of Reproductive Medicine, 45*, 936-938.

Gonder-Frederick, L.A. (2001). Hypoglycemia. In M.J. Franz (Ed.), *A Core Curriculum of Diabetes Education: Diabetes Management Therapies* (4th ed.) (pp. 231-260). Chicago: American Association of Diabetes Educators.

Harris, M.I., Flegal, K.M., Cowie, C.C., Eberhardt, M.S., Goldstein, D.E., Little, R.R., Weidmeyer, H. & Byrd-Holt, D.D. (1998). Prevalence of diabetes, impaired fasting glucose and impaired glucose tolerance in U.S. adults. The Third National Health and Nutrition Examination Survey, 1988-1994. *Diabetes Care, 21*, 518-524.

Heller, S.R. & Cryer, P.E. (1991). Reduced neuroendocrine and symptomatic responses to subsequent hypoglycemia after one episode of hypoglycemia in non-diabetic humans. *Diabetes, 40*, 223-226.

Holing, E.V., Beyer, C.S., Brown, Z.A. & Connell, F.A. (1998). Why don't women with diabetes plan their pregnancies? *Diabetes Care, 21*, 889-895.

Homko, C.J. (1998). Gestational diabetes: A screening and management update. *Advance for Nurse Practitioners, 6*, 59-63.

Homko, C.J. & Jornsay, D. (2001). Pregnancy: Preconception to postpartum. In M.J. Franz (Ed.), *A Core Curriculum of Diabetes Education: Diabetes in the Life Cycle and Research* (4th ed.) (pp. 33-69). Chicago: American Association of Diabetes Educators.

Homko, C.J. & Khandelwal, M. (1996). Glucose monitoring and insulin therapy in pregnancy. *Obstetrics and Gynecology Clinics of North America, 23*, 47-74.

Ilic, S., Jovanovic, L. & Jeng, L. (2000). Continuous glucose monitoring identifies postprandial hyperglycemia missed by standard glucose monitoring in gestational diabetes. *Diabetes, 49*, (Suppl. 1), A443.

Jornsay, D.L. (1998). Continuous subcutaneous insulin infusion (CSII) therapy during pregnancy. *Diabetes Spectrum, 11*, 26-32, 51.

Jovanovic, L. (2000). *Medical management of pregnancy complicated by diabetes mellitus.* Alexandria, VA: American Diabetes Association.

Jovanovic, L., Ilic, S., Pettitt, D.J., Hugo, K., Gutierrez, M., Bowsher, R.R. & Bastyr, E.J., III. (1999). Metabolic and immunologic effects of insulin lispro in gestational diabetes. *Diabetes Care, 22*, 1422-1427.

Jungheim, K. & Koschinsky, T. (2001). Risky delay of hypoglycemia detection by glucose monitoring at the arm. *Diabetes Care, 24*, 1303-1306.

Karter, A.J., Ackerson, L.M., Darbinian, J.A., D'Agostino, R.B., Jr., Ferrara, A., Liu, J. & Selby, J.V. (2001). Self-monitoring of blood glucose levels and glycemic control: The Northern California Kaiser Permanente Diabetes Register. *American Journal of Medicine, 111*, 1-9.

Kemball, M.L., McIver, C., Milner, R.D., Nourse, C.H., Schiff, D. & Tiernan, J.R. (1970). Neonatal hypoglycemia in infants of diabetic mothers given sulphonylurea drugs in pregnancy. *Archives of Disease in Childhood, 45*, 696-670.

Kendrick, J.M. (1999). Diabetes mellitus in pregnancy. In L.K. Mandeville & N.H. Troiano (Eds.), *AWHONN's high risk and critical care intrapartum nursing* (pp. 224-254). Philadelphia: Lippincott, Williams & Wilkins.

Kendrick, J.M. (2001). Diabetes. In K.R. Simpson & P. Crehan (Eds.), *AWHONN'S Perinatal Nursing* (2nd ed.) (pp. 219-235). Philadelphia: Lippincott, Williams & Wilkins.

Kent, L.A., Gill, G.V. & Williams, G. (1994). Mortality and outcome of patients with brittle diabetes and recurrent ketoacidosis. *Lancet, 344*, 778-781.

Kimmerle, R., Zass, R.P., Cupisti, S., Somville, T., Bender, R., Pawloski, B. & Berger, M. (1995). Pregnancies in women with diabetic nephropathy: Long-term outcome for mother and child. *Diabetologia, 38*, 227-235.

Kitzmiller, J.L., Main, E., Ward, B., Theiss, T. & Peterson, D.L. (1999). Insulin lispro and the development of proliferative diabetic retinopathy in pregnancy. *Diabetes Care, 22*, 874-875.

Kjos, S.L. (2000). Postpartum care of the woman with diabetes. *Clinical Obstetrics and Gynecology, 43*, 75-86.

Kjos, S.L., Henry, O., Lee, R.M., Buchanan, T.A. & Mishell, D.R., Jr. (1993). The effect of lactation on glucose and lipid metabolism in women with recent gestational diabetes. *Obstetrics and Gynecology, 82*, 451-455.

Kjos, S.L., Peters, R.K., Xiang, A., Thomas, D., Schaefer, U. & Buchanan, T.A. (1998). Contraception and the risk of type 2 diabetes in Latina women with prior gestational diabetes mellitus. *JAMA, 280*, 533-538.

Lamar, M.E., Kuehl, T.J., Cooney, A.T., Gayle, L.J., Holleman, S. & Allen, S.R. (1999). Jelly beans as an alternative to a 50-gram glucose beverage for gestational diabetes screening. *American Journal of Obstetrics and Gynecology, 181*, 1154-1157.

Landon, M.B. (2000). Obstetric management of pregnancies complicated by diabetes mellitus. *Clinical Obstetrics and Gynecology, 43*, 65-74.

Langan, S.J., Dreary, I.J., Hepburn, D.A. & Frier, B. M. (1991). Cumulative cognitive impairment following recurrent severe hypoglycemia in adult patients with insulin-treated diabetes mellitus. *Diabetologia, 34*, 333-343.

Langer, N. & Langer, O. (1998). Pre-existing diabetics: Relationships between glycemic control and emotional status in pregnancy. *Journal of Maternal Fetal Medicine, 7*, 257-263.

Langer, N. & Langer, O. (2000). Comparison of pregnancy mood profiles in gestational diabetes and preexisting diabetes. *Diabetes Educator, 26*, 667-672.

Langer, O. (2000). Management of gestational diabetes. *Clincal Obstetrics and Gynecology, 43*, 337-344.

Langer, O., Conway, D.L., Berkus, M.D., Xenaki, E.M. & Gonzales, O. (2000). A comparison of glyburide and insulin in women with gestational diabetes mellitus. *New England Journal of Medicine, 343*, 1134-1138.

Logan, M. (1993). Lower extremity problems. In V. Peragallo-Dittko, K. Godley & J. Meyer (Eds.), *A Core Curriculum of Diabetes Education* (pp. 687-697). Chicago: Port City Press.

Lustman, P.J., Anderson, R.J., Freedland, K.E., de Groot, M., Carney, R.M. & Clouse, R.E. (2000). Depression and poor glycemic control: Meta-analytic review of the literature. *Diabetes Care, 23*, 934-942.

Major, C.A., de Veciana, M., Weeks, J. & Morgan, M.A. (1998). Recurrence of gestational diabetes: Who is at risk? *American Journal of Obstetrics & Gynecology, 179*, 1038-1042.

March of Dimes. (1999). *Bereavement kit.* White Plains, NY: Author.

March of Dimes. (2002). *Eating for two.* White Plains, NY: Author.

Marcus, A.O. & Fernandez, M.P. (1996). Insulin pump therapy: acceptable alternative to injection therapy. *Postgraduate Medicine, 99*(3), 125-132, 142-144.

Matthews, D.R. (1999). The natural history diabetes-related complications: The UKPDS experience. *Diabetes Obesity and Metabolism, 1*(Suppl. 2), 7-13.

McGarraugh, G. (2001). Glucose monitoring at the arm. Letter to the editor. *Diabetes Care, 24*, 1304-1306.

Mokdad, A.H., Bowman, B.A., Ford, E.S., Vinicor, F., Marks, J.S. & Koplan, J.P. (2001). The continuing epidemics of obesity and diabetes in the United States. *JAMA, 286*(10), 1195-200.

Mokdad, A.H., Ford, E.S., Bowman, B.A., Nelson, D.E., Engelgau, M.M., Vinicor, F. & Marks, J.S. (2001). The continuing increase of diabetes in the U.S. *Diabetes Care, 24*, 412.

Mokdad, A.H., Ford, E.S., Bowman, B.A., Nelson, D.E., Engelgau, M.M., Vinicor, F. & Marks, J.S. (2000). Diabetes trends in the U.S.: 1990-1998. *Diabetes Care, 23*(9), 1278-83.

Mokdad, A.H., Serdula, M.K., Dietz, W.H., Bowman, B.A., Marks, J.S. & Koplan, J.P. (1999). The spread of the obesity epidemic in the United States, 1991-1998. *JAMA, 282*(16), 1519-22.

Moore, T.R. (1999). Diabetes in pregnancy. In R.K. Creasy & R.A. Resnik (Eds.), *Maternal Fetal Medicine* (4th ed.) (pp. 964-995). Philadelphia: W.B. Saunders.

Moos, M.K. (2003). *Preconception health promotion: A focus for women's wellness.* White Plains, NY: March of Dimes.

Mulooly, C.A. (2001). Exercise. In M.J. Franz (Ed.), *A Core Curriculum of Diabetes Education: Diabetes Management Therapies* (4th ed.) (pp. 57-88). Chicago: American Association of Diabetes Educators.

National Institute of Diabetes and Digestive and Kidney Diseases (NIDDK). (1999). *Gastroparesis and diabetes.* NIH Publication #99-4348. Bethesda, MD: Author.

Nelson, A., Hatcher, R.A., Zieman, M., Watt, A., Darney, P.D. & Creuinin, M.D. (2000). Managing contraception: Millennium edition 2000-2001 (3rd ed.). Dawsonville, GA: Bridging the Gap Foundation.

Passanza, C.E. (2001). Diabetes update: Monitor options. *RN, 64*, 36-42.

Pedersen, J., Pedersen, L.M. & Andersen, B. (1974). Assessors of fetal perinatal mortality in diabetic pregnancy. Analysis of 1,332 pregnancies in the Copenhagen series, 1946-1972. *Diabetes, 23*, 302-305.

Peragallo-Dittko, V. (2001). Monitoring. In M.J. Franz (Ed.), *A Core Curriculum of Diabetes Education: Diabetes Management Therapies* (4th ed.) (pp. 153-172). Chicago: American Association of Diabetes Educators.

Perez-Bravo, F., Carrasco, E., Gutierez-Lopez, M.D., Martinez, M.T., Lopez, G. & de los Rios, M.G. (1996). Genetic predisposition and environmental factors leading to the development of insulin dependent diabetes mellitus in Chilean children. *Journal of Molecular Medicine, 74*, 105-109.

Perucchini, D., Fischer, U., Spinas, G.A., Huch, R., Huch, A. & Lehmann, R. (1999). Using fasting plasma glucose concentrations to screen for gestational diabetes mellitus: Prospective population based study. *BMJ, 319*, 812-815.

Pettitt, D.J., Forman, M.R., Hanson, R.L., Knowler, W.C. & Bennett, P.H. (1997). Breastfeeding and incidence of non-insulin dependent diabetes mellitus in Pima Indians. *Lancet, 350*, 166-168.

Peyrot, M. & Rubin, R.R. (1997). Levels and risks of depression and anxiety symptomatology among diabetic adults. *Diabetes Care, 20*, 585-590.

Pouwer, F., Snoek, F.J., Van Der Ploeg, H.M., Ader, H.J. & Heine, R.J. (2001). Monitoring psychological well-being in outpatients with diabetes: Effects on mood, HbA (1c) and the patient's evaluation of the quality of diabetes care. *Diabetes Care, 24*, 1929-1935.

Ramer, L. & Frank, B. (2001). *Pregnancy: Psychosocial perspectives* (3rd ed.). White Plains, NY: March of Dimes.

Ramin, K.D. (1999). Diabetic ketoacidosis in pregnancy. *Obstetrics and Gynecology Clinics of North America, 26*, 481-488.

Ratner, R.E. (2001). Pathophysiology of diabetes disease state. In M.J. Franz (Ed.), *A Core Curriculum of Diabetes Education: Diabetes and Complications* (4th ed.) (pp. 1-18). Chicago: American Association of Diabetes Educators.

Reece, E.A. & Homko, C.J. (1994). Infant of the diabetic mother. *Seminars in Perinatology, 18*, 459-469.

Reece, E.A., Leguizamon, G. & Homko, C. (1998). Pregnancy performance and outcomes associated with diabetic nephropathy. *American Journal of Perinatology, 15*, 413-421.

Rosenn, B.M. & Miodovnik, M. (2000). Medical complications of diabetes mellitus in pregnancy. *Clinical Obstetrics and Gynecology, 43*, 17-31.

Rosenn, B.M., Miodovnik, M., Holcberg, G., Khoury, J.C. & Siddiqi, T.A. (1995). Hypoglycemia: The price of intensive insulin therapy for pregnant women with insulin dependent diabetes mellitus. *Obstetrics and Gynecology, 85*, 417-422.

Rosenn, B.M., Miodovnik, M., Khoury, J. & Siddiqi, T.A. (1996). Counterregulatory responses to hypoglycemia in pregnant women with insulin dependent diabetes mellitus. *Obstetrics and Gynecology, 87*, 568-574.

Rubin, R.R. & Napora, J.P. (2001). Psychosocial assessment. In M.J. Franz (Ed.), *A Core Curriculum of Diabetes Education: Diabetes Education and Program Management* (4th ed.) (pp. 24-64). Chicago: American Association of Diabetes Educators.

Schwartz, R. & Teramo, K.A. (2000). Effects of diabetic pregnancy on the fetus and newborn, *Seminars in Perinatology, 24*, 120-135.

Silverman, B.L., Rizzo, T.A., Cho, N.H. & Metzger, B.E. (1998). Long-term effects of the intrauterine environment, The Northwestern University Diabetes in Pregnancy Center. *Diabetes Care, 2* (Suppl. 2), B142-49.

Star, J. & Carpenter, M.W. (1998). The effect of pregnancy on the natural history of diabetic retinopathy and nephropathy. *Clinics in Perinatology, 25*, 887-916.

Stevenson, D.K. (1987). Bilirubin metabolism in the infant of the diabetic mother. An overview. In S.G. Gabbe (Ed.), *Infant of the diabetic mother. Report of the 93rd Conference on Pediatric Research* (pp. 109-117). Columbus, OH: Ross Laboratories.

Trief, P.M., Himes, C.L., Orendorff, R. & Weinstock, R.S. (2001). The marital relationship and psychosocial adaptation and glycemic control of individuals with diabetes. *Diabetes Care, 24*, 1384-1389.

Vargo, L.E. & Trotter, C.W. (1998). *The premature infant: Nursing assessment and management.* White Plains, NY: March of Dimes.

Vinicor, R. (2001). Macrovascular disease. In M.J. Franz (Ed.), *A Core Curriculum of Diabetes Education: Diabetes and Complications* (4th ed.) (pp. 99-122). Chicago: American Association of Diabetes Educators.

Windebank, A.J. & Feldman, E.L. (2001). Diabetes and the nervous system. In M.J. Aminoff (Ed.), *Neurology and General Medicine* (pp. 341-364). New York: Churchill Livingstone.

White, P. (1949). Pregnancy complicating diabetes. *American Journal of Medicine*, *7*, 609-616.

Whiteman, V.E., Homko, C.J. & Reece, E.A. (1996). Management of hypoglycemia and diabetic ketoacidosis in pregnancy. *Obstetrics and Gynecology Clinics in North America*, *23*, 87-107.

American Academy of Pediatrics (AAP) & The American College of Obstetricians and Gynecologists. (2002). *Guidelines for perinatal care* (5th ed.). Elk Grove Village, IL: AAP.

Presents guidelines for perinatal health care providers on preconception care, care during and after birth, data documentation and financing. Defines levels of care in terms of facilities, equipment and personnel from obstetric and pediatric standpoints, including regionalization of perinatal and pediatric care, substance abuse, domestic violence and obstetric complications.

Bakewell-Sachs, S. Shaw, V.D. & Tashman, A.L. (1997). *Assessment of risk in the term newborn.* White Plains, NY: March of Dimes.

Provides information on assessment of newborn infectious or metabolic disorders and physiologic adaptation to extrauterine life, including gestational age assessment, physical assessment and newborn behavior patterns. Discusses nursing management during the early newborn period, including identification of risk factors, assessment, monitoring, intervention during hospitalization and post-discharge follow-up.

Biancuzzo, M. (1994). *Breastfeeding the healthy newborn.* White Plains, NY: March of Dimes.

Identifies biological, psychological and sociocultural factors that influence success for breastfeeding mothers and their full-term newborns. Describes effective communication techniques to help mothers breastfeed. Includes physical assessment skills and clinical management strategies to prevent and solve common breastfeeding problems.

Breedlove, G.K. & Schorfheide, A.M. (2001). *Adolescent pregnancy* (2nd ed.). White Plains, NY: March of Dimes.

Follows a community health promotion model of prevention and intervention, including discussion of adolescent development, risk-taking behavior and peer influence (primary prevention); management of adolescent pregnancy through the maternity cycle (secondary prevention); and promotion of health youth restoration and risk reduction (tertiary prevention). Presents current trends, research and policy issues.

Deacon, J. & O'Neill, P. (2000). *A core curriculum for neonatal intensive care nursing* (2nd ed.). Philadelphia: W.B. Saunders.

Provides guidelines for intensive nursing care of the neonate. Defines neonatal conditions and gives information on incidence, etiology, pathophysiology, clinical presentation, diagnosis and management.

Dowling, D., Danner, S.C., & Coffey, P.M. (1997). *Breastfeeding the infant with special needs.* White Plains, NY: March of Dimes.

Addresses techniques for supporting the breastfeeding dyad when the infant has special needs. Describes hands-on, clinical support techniques for breastfeeding premature infants and infants with cleft lip and palate, neurological disorders and cardiac disorders.

Franz, M.J. (2001). *A core curriculum for diabetes education* (4th ed.). Chicago: Port City Press.

Includes information on care of pregnant women from preconception to postpartum and care and education of women with gestational diabetes.

Jovanovic, L. (2000). *Medical management of pregnancy complicated by diabetes* (3rd ed.). Alexandria, VA: American Diabetes Association.

Guides the care of pregnant women with pregestational and gestational diabetes from preconception to postpartum. Serves as protocol development for physicians, nurses and others caring for pregnant women with diabetes. Includes information on psychological impact of diabetes; medical nutrition therapy; insulin therapy; self-management; maternal-fetal antepartum surveillance; screening, diagnosis and intervention for gestational diabetes; and neonatal care.

Mattson, S. & Smith, J.E. (1999). *Core curriculum for maternal-newborn nursing*. Philadelphia: W.B. Saunders.

A reference for nurses who care for women and newborns. Presents information on nursing assessment, diagnosis, intervention and evaluation. Describes fetal growth and development, maternal-fetal well-being, intrapartum and postpartum care and care of the normal newborn. Describes nursing care of pregnant women with complications, including medical disorders, trauma in pregnancy, surgery during pregnancy, substance abuse, infections, hemorrhagic disorders and postpartum complication. Discusses complications of the newborn period.

Moos, M.K. (2003). *Preconception health promotion: A focus for women's wellness*. White Plains, NY: March of Dimes.

Addresses the importance of nurses in promoting preconception wellness, updates information and research on health promotion content and explores opportunities for providing health information to prospective parents. Explores the rationale behind pre-pregnancy health, provides guidance on preconception risk identification and outlines approaches to promoting preconception wellness.

Ramer, L. & Frank, B. (2001). *Pregnancy: Psychosocial perspectives* (3rd ed.). White Plains, NY: March of Dimes.

Focuses on common and expected transitions experienced by families during pregnancy. Presents childbearing in a family-centered, wellness-oriented, culturally meaningful context. Considers individual experiences, personal adaptations and adjustments in interpersonal relationships.

Vargo, L.E. & Trotter, C.W. (1998). *The premature infant: Nursing assessment and management*. White Plains, NY: March of Dimes.

Addresses the pathyophysiology of respiratory, cardiovascular, immunologic and neurologic problems commonly facing the premature infant in the neonatal intensive care unit. Discusses prevention of prematurity, respiratory distress syndrome, bronchopulmonary dysplasia, apnea of prematurity, hypotension, patent ductus arteriosis, sepsis and intraventricular hemorrhage. Describes treatments, interventions and nursing implications.